Wellness East and West

Wellness
East and West

———

**Achieving Optimum Health
through Integrative Medicine**

Kathleen F. Phalen

JOURNEY EDITIONS
BOSTON • TOKYO

Publisher's Note: The purpose of this book is to educate. It is sold with the understanding that the author and Journey Editions shall have neither liability nor responsibility for any injury caused or alleged to be caused directly or indirectly by the information contained in this book. The adoption and application of the material offered in this book is at the reader's discretion and sole responsibility. While every effort has been made to ensure its accuracy, the book's contents should not be construed as medical advice. Each person's health needs are unique. To obtain recommendations appropriate to your particular situation, please consult a qualified health care provider.

First paperback edition published in 1999 by Journey Editions, an imprint of Periplus Editions (HK) Ltd., with editorial offices at 153 Milk Street, Boston, Massachusetts 02109.

Library of Congress Cataloging-in-Publication Data

Phalen, Kathleen F.
Wellness East and West : Achieving Optimum Health through
Integrative Medicine / Kathleen F. Phalen. — 1st ed.
p. cm.
Includes bibliographical references (p.).
ISBN 1-885203-61-6
1. Alternative medicine. I. Title.
R733.P44 1998
615.5 — dc21   98-8672
CIP

DISTRIBUTED BY

NORTH AMERICA
Charles E. Tuttle Co., Inc.
RR 1 Box 231-5
North Clarendon, VT 05759
Tel: (802) 773-8930
Tel: (800) 526-2778

CANADA
Raincoast Books
8680 Cambie Street
Vancouver, British Columbia V6P 6M9
Tel: (604) 323-7100
Fax: (604) 323-2600

JAPAN
Tuttle Shokai Ltd.
1-21-13, Seki
Tama-ku, Kawasaki-shi
Kanagawa-ken 214, Japan
Tel: (044) 833-0225
Fax: (044) 822-0413

SOUTHEAST ASIA
Berkeley Books Pte. Ltd.
5 Little Road #08-01
Singapore 536983
Tel: (65) 280-3320
Fax: (65) 280-6290

First paperback edition
07 06 05 04 03 02 01 00 99   10 9 8 7 6 5 4 3 2 1

TEXT DESIGN BY JILL WINITZER
PRINTED IN THE UNITED STATES OF AMERICA

To each of us as we journey toward wellness.
Look for the beating of the human heart,
the beauty of the universe, and the healer within.

Acknowledgments

There are not enough pages to thank everyone who so generously contributed to the creation of this book. Hundreds of patient and practioner interviews and countless individuals who let me sit in and observe their care and treatment. Researchers who so graciously shared the details of their findings. And most of all my family, friends and dogs, who cooked me a meal or went with me for a walk in the mountains just to help me get through this time-consuming process. I send out all the loving energies of the universe to everyone who assisted me on my path. There are some people I would like to mention because of their considerable contribution to *Wellness East and West*.

My daughter Johanna, my granddaughter Malia, my grandson Blaine, and my son-in-law Kevin for their daily support, meals, love, and deliveries of wood, not to mention all the photocopying and reading Johanna did. My daughter Rebecca for her enduring support, editing, love, and encouragement. To Emilie and Ivy, my golden retriever and chocolate lab for giving up their walks on some days and just staying by my side giving me unconditional love. To my parents, Ken and Lois Pasch, for loving me, accepting my eccentric ways, and pushing me to finish. To Kathy Balog, my sister in spirit. To Doug Schneider, Faye Satterly, and Stephanie Stapleton for loving me in spite of my unavailability. To Denny Deysher, the best newspaper editor ever. To my agent, Nina Graybill, for her insight, and to my editors at Tuttle Publishing. And to the following practitioners and patients for their incredible guidance and support. Especially George Wedemeyer, Robert Duggan, and Carolyn Jaffe, who showed me the heart behind the treatment. Also Claire Cassidy, Sandra McLanahan, Tricia Yu, Jody Forman, Peter Bower, Cindy Janechild, Rebecca Phalen, Lee Felton, Rae Ellison, Bernie Siegel, Pali DeLevitt, Paul Olko, Jacki Rooke, Howard Moffett, Rebecca Hotzmiller, Elizabeth Zintle (now deceased), and Hebrew Watson.

Contents

Foreword

Wellness is a meeting point of many different facets of our life: the scientific, the interpersonal, the way we eat, the way we sleep, the way we deal with our emotions. Healing involves interpersonal relationships between individuals and those whom they invite to be in healing relationships with them.

It is clear that we are moving from a world in which we look to experts in health care to make decisions for us to a world in which we have recovered our ability, as individuals, families, and communities, to heal ourselves and to make the advice and skills of the "experts" supplemental to our reliance on the innate human ability to heal. We are in a period of redefining the idea of health and recovering the awareness that a life well lived is characterized by the ability to cope with suffering and to live life in the presence of death. We are also coming to recognize that the expectation of living life without pain and suffering is unrealistic, and that human cultures cannot afford to go on believing otherwise.

Kathleen Phalen starts from the perspective of a journalist reporting on emerging phenomena in our culture. She gives us a book different from others in its scope and presentation.

Here you will find the stories of many individuals—stories that most readers will recognize. You will also find lists of illnesses and suggested remedies, as well as new ways of thinking. Uniquely, Kathleen points out the possibilities confronting each individual as he or she copes with various symptoms, and she brings to her presentation the awareness that symptoms may be teachers and guides that each of us and our practitioners must interpret in a different way. And she also offers a solid presentation of the available research and the relationships that exist between mainstream researchers at the

National Institutes of Health, physicians, and practitioners of alternative medicine, as well as an understanding of the enormous drive of the American public to recover something that has been lost but that was well known to our ancestors.

There are answers. And when you find an answer, you will also find another question. *Wellness East and West* is a wonderful blend of factual material, possible options, creative thinking, and personal stories. Mostly I appreciate the personal passion that I witnessed in Kathleen as she went through the process of writing this book, her excitement and passion about the stories of the many individuals with whom she spoke, her sense that something new was happening and awakening, and her craving to find a way to share a complex mix of old and new ideas.

> —*Robert Duggan, MAc, MA, DiplAc (NCCA),*
> *president and cofounder, Traditional Acupuncture*
> *Institute, Columbia, Maryland*
> *In 1994 he was appointed chairman of the Maryland*
> *State Board of Acupuncture and now serves on many*
> *national health care advisory panels including programs*
> *for the NIH.*

Introduction

Somewhere between the diaphanous folds of living, loving, grieving, and dying lies the hidden truth of healing. But much like the early morning's mist gently rising above the dewy ground, its simplicity eludes us. We reach out, but often in our desperation we try too hard, and the answer scatters among the tubes, needles, drugs, and heroic measures. Begging for life and healing at any cost becomes our mantra. But there are those who in recent years have asked, *why?* And while the answers are as individual as those exploring new healing avenues, common threads emerge: the need to examine our own beliefs about healing; the desire to connect physically and spiritually with healers; the quest to simplify; and the willingness to try alternative paths. This book illustrates how ancient Eastern remedies are being integrated with Western treatments and offers an overview of the transition that is gradually occurring in our nation's health care treatment options. It offers insight into not only patients' feelings and experiences but also practitioners'. And perhaps most of all, it shows that many people have the desire to meet somewhere in the middle.

This journey has been one of excitement, agony, discovery, and wonder. Having worked for many years as a health reporter and writer, I was very familiar with conventional Western medicine and its practitioners. I have seen the good and the bad over time. And because of this I was often disillusioned with a system that I believed was seriously failing those seeking help and guidance. This book has changed my mind. It is a book about hope. It is about love. It is about healing, not curing.

This project began when I was given a newspaper assignment to cover a story on an acupuncturist. My editors pushed me to verify all her credentials. This was in 1995, a time when people in Reading, a city in south central Pennsylvania, didn't often hear about alternative healing or such crazy ideas as moxibustion—the Chinese practice of burning *moxa* (mugwort herb) over an acupuncture point—or cupping—the Chinese practice of placing heated jars on the back to help restore the flow of *qi* (the body's energy). To further legitimize the article, I asked the acupuncturist to have a few patients available for me to interview.

I arrived at her office on a cold February day. It was icy, and I was certain no one would be there. Running a few minutes late, I flew into the front waiting area where I was struck by the number of faces meeting my astonished gaze. There were grandmothers and farmers and young people and businessmen, all there to tell me their tales of recovery. I could hardly keep pace. But all the stories had a common thread. The patients had a tremendous loyalty to Carolyn Jaffe, their acupuncturist, because they felt she listened to and loved them. She had helped free them of conditions that had plagued many of them for twenty-five or thirty years. They spoke of getting off all their medications, of getting off the breathing machine, of being able to work or play tennis or just be well. I have to admit I was overwhelmed by all the people who showed up, and finally I had to tell Carolyn, "No more people."

The story ran several weeks later in the Lifestyle section of the paper, and within twenty-four hours I personally had received nearly a hundred phone calls at the newsroom. "Do you think she can help my arthritis?" "Does that help headaches?" "I have cancer. Do you think she can help me?" Simultaneously, Carolyn's phone was ringing off the hook, and she was booked with appointments for nearly six months. Not to mention the Lifestyle editor, who got calls similar to the ones I received. It was obvious; people were searching for more. So I began researching the topic. Now, three years later, I bring you *Wellness East and West*. It is a compilation of the information I have gathered from around the country, of my conversations with practitioners and patients, and a limited survey of what's happening with research, the National Institutes of Health, with insurance companies, and in anecdotal studies. This is only the beginning. I am only barely scratching the surface of the countless changes and improvements happening across the nation.

Although I write about the Eastern and Western approaches to treatment and how many people have found ways to blend the two, my greatest discovery was the unifying force between the medical traditions of the East and the West. It is a meeting in the middle, in love and compassion. I learned that our healing comes from within, and that we must find ways to simplify and love ourselves. Then the force of love will radiate out from our own center.

I think in many ways that when we are sick, we tend to get lost in all the technology and drugs. Our health care dilemma could be less complex if we could rid ourselves of the barriers to treatment. And while some of the blame for these barriers can be laid at the feet of the third-party payers (insurers, managed care, health maintenance organizations) and the regulators (like the Food and Drug Administration), some of the burden is our own. We are too stressed, we eat all the wrong foods, we isolate ourselves from others, and we have been persuaded to believe that there is something inherently wrong with natural physiological processes and life cycles. Menopause is as natural for women as puberty or childbirth, yet many women fear its onset. Death is seen as a failure of our doctors. But we all will die. We need to understand that there can be healing even in disease. Granted, Eastern and Western therapies cannot provide a cure for everything. And sometimes learning to live, even with disease, is part of healing. The choice is ours; to die while living or to live each day in grace, with ease, seeing the beauty and wonder in all that is ours. We need to reclaim memories of lying in the tall grass on a summer's afternoon and watching the clouds transform from dinosaurs to witches to angels. Let's recapture the burning pleasure of doing just about nothing, remembering the days when we would go to the pond's edge to catch frogs and etch our names in the red clay or make mudpies topped with flaming dandelions. At a time when our legs were still short enough to keep us close to the ground, we knew how to live. The answer lies somewhere between here and those dreamy summer's days. It's as individual as there are people on this earth.

We need to start following our heart. To make loving, living choices. It's not an us and them thing, it's an us thing. We need to live more simply: to enjoy the intensity of a shared smile; the beauty of autumn's changing hues or the ethereal image of winter's frozen flakes performing a gentle waltz in the incandescent rays of the city lights. Beauty is everywhere: inside and out. It's in the city, in the mountains, in the desert. We need to take the time and look for it in our hearts, in the face of a homeless person, in a dog's gentle kiss, in the wondrous giggle of a child.

Blessings of the universe,
Kathleen F. Phalen

ONE

The Birth of Integrative Medicine

"The utmost in the art of healing can be achieved when there is unity. When the minds of the people are closed and wisdom is locked out, they remain tied to disease. Yet their feelings and desires should be investigated and made known, their wishes and ideas should be followed, and then it becomes apparent that those who have attained spirit and energy are flourishing and prosperous, while those perish who lose their spirit and energy."

—From the *Nei Ching Su Wen*

CENTURIES OF HEALING WISDOM

We are certain the cure will be in the next pill, the next prayer, the next visit to the doctor. And in many ways we are not alone. The search for a cure has led even the crustiest of souls to the far reaches of the earth—to the healing waters of Lourdes, to an appointment with the surgeon's scalpel, to the shaman's medicine bag, to the acupuncturist's needles, to taking transfusions of another person's blood, to exposing ourselves to deadly gamma rays, or to taking addicting pain deadeners. Sometimes it seems we would do just about anything to find the golden cure.

Ancient cultures were no exception. People in the earliest civilizations suffered from chronic and life-threatening conditions—very similar to today's ills—and they, too, searched for remedies to stop the pain and extend life. Those ancient peoples knew much more about tending each other, the living and the dying. Their connection to the heavens and the earth wasn't complicated by 156 selections on satellite television or the horrors of the evening news, and, while they often faced the harsh realities of nature's elements with fewer protections, their essence was not lost in a lonely world where everything happens too fast. They listened to themselves, to their neighbors, and to the hearts of their ancestors.

In their less complicated lives, they were not spared the pain of living—the grieving, the loss, the sickness. And as primitive scratchings on dampened cave walls indicate, even in the earliest of times man suffered from headaches, chronic conditions, and sexually transmitted diseases. Archeological digs have revealed prehistoric art showing that holes were bored through human skulls to relieve pressure. Neolithic man endured the daily pain of osteoarthritis. There are the calcified remains of parasitic eggs known to cause the tropical disease schistosomiasis in Egyptian mummies.[1] And petrified syphilitic skulls, dating back prior to Columbus's historic journey to the New World, have been uncovered in North America.[2]

Just like the diseases and the physical and mental ills that existed long before us, the natural impulse to stop the suffering, to find a better way, is nothing new, even though some try to lay claim to this innovative thinking. Today bulletin boards at trendy health food stores contain messages of healing—the new blue-green algae, the latest inner child healing workshop, or the spiritually centered ads about reconnecting with nature—tacked to their cork surfaces with multicolored pushpins. Or better yet, there are tear-off phone numbers so that the desperate can call for help twenty-four hours a day. Hip, pop-culture magazines are filled with the claims of new life from New Age healers. On the Internet you can get a *reiki* consultation, and herbs to kill your bad breath and the dog's at the same time. The secrets behind these dramatic breakthroughs and discoveries about stopping the pain and healing our bodies, our odors, our relationships, as well as the universe around us, can be ours with just a credit card number.

What we often don't realize in our search for healing is that many of the concepts and theories that are being touted these days have been around since a time when it was OK to believe in myth, a time when legend was passed from generation to generation. Finding a way to wellness dates back to an era when legend could become reality. Today we have come to a threshold in which we understand what our ancestors perhaps took for granted—that healing is everyone's business and responsibility, and that it is something that involves our understanding and active participation.

The healing traditions of our neighbors in the East, which go back centuries of generations, are steeped in parables and evidence a connection between health, spirituality, and the cosmos. In China, Han dynasty tombs preserved fragments of exemplary medical information, which, according to legend and generations of believers, were first penned by the mythical Yellow Emperor, who is said to have reigned from 2696 B.C. to 2598 B.C. Beginning with conversations between the emperor and his physician, the *Nei Ching Su Wen,* or *The Yellow Emperor's Classic of Internal Medicine,* establishes the concept that supports the need for a positive doctor-patient relationship. With information on drugs, surgery, medical theory, spirituality, life force, the balance of yin and yang, the five elements (wood, fire, metal, air, and water), and the four seasons of healing, this comprehensive record remains a main source of guidance for many Eastern cultures and health practitioners today.[3]

Sumerian cuneiform clay tablets, dating from somewhere around 2500 B.C., tell tales of illness and list the details of medicinal plants and animal parts prescribed for treating the ills of the time. Historians are unable to determine whether the Sumerians actually discovered these healing arts or whether the concepts were borrowed from other cultures. Many of these medicinal remedies were divided into organic and inorganic categories, with plant remedies such as figs, dates, anise, jasmine, juniper, coriander, caraway, and willow.[4] Passing this legacy of knowledge and healing on to the Babylonians, the Sumerians set in motion a generational chain of curative information that formed the rudimentary foundations of Western medicine. The embryonic Sumerian teachings traveled history's course, crossing lands and time. Eventually uncovered by Egypt's Pharaohs, these healing arts evolved to yet another level. And as writings preserved in papyrus tell us, elaborate theories explaining the cause of physical ills took on dramatic proportions. The Egyptians believed that sickness originated in the supernatural realm, and that healing took place on the physical and spiritual planes.

As the discoveries of healers became paradigms for their culture, the integral rhythm of contrasting internal and external forces was seen as reigning over the body. Chinese healers set forth the delicate balance of yin and yang: yin, the feminine force of darkness, night, moon, moistness, quiet, and earth; yang, the masculine force of light, sun, day, dryness, fire, heat, heaven, noise, and function. Yin, representing the internal, descends; yang, the external, ascends. It was believed, and is still believed today, that each of the body's organs has an element of yin and yang, and that health is achieved by keeping the two in balance.

Similar to Chinese healers, Greek physicians looked at the nature of disease as sets of opposites: hot and cold, moist and dry. They also described and diagnosed illness based on the four humors—blood, phlegm, and black and yellow bile. The thread that binds these ancient beliefs is the theory that a vital life force, when kept in balance, can ward off disease. And whether it is called *qi* (Chinese, pronounced *chee*), *lung* (Tibetan, pronounced *loong*), or *prana*, meaning breath, maintaining or restoring balance was the physician's secret for preventing disease.[5]

Ancient healers developed an intimate bond with their patients; they believed, above all, that nothing must be done to injure the patient. Whether taking a history, feeling the pulse, or gauging the heat of the body, each practiced the gentle art of his or her respective beliefs. Medical advice, even in more primitive times, paralleled much of what the adventurous preach today—diet, exercise, prevention. The Chinese, much like the Tibetans, talked openly about combining tranquil, moderate exercise with seasonal diets, stressing the importance of a serene mind. They believed that it is better to prevent illness than to try to cure it once it occurs—a concept we're just getting around to understanding in this modern age of Western medicine. We've certainly made a lot of progress in the last two thousand years!

The use of plants and herbs was already highly developed in many cultures many centuries ago. Thriving pharmacopoeias were produced in China, Egypt, and Greece. The Chinese, who were using acupuncture in addition to herbs, massage, and gentle exercise, had delineated points on the body that could be needled or cauterized to cure or alleviate pain associated with most ailments. Historians indicate that the Chinese may have filtered water and prescribed boiling water and eating hot dishes as a means of avoiding infection.[6] Because Egyptians actively engaged in embalming the dead, they began to learn the delicate intricacies of the human anatomy. Egyptians and Greeks used herbs and foods to balance the humors, often using St. John's Wort, yarrow, and plantain to heal wounds and ward off illness. And whether Chinese, Egyptian, or Greek, disease prevention teachings, along with suggestions for keeping the body in balance, were a major component of these early beliefs.

During medieval times and even later, setbacks were not uncommon. Wars, cultural revolutions, plagues, malnutrition, and rampant disease left many victims in their wake. Keeping pace with the turbulence and magnitude of disease and death was challenging for physicians, at best. And in the 1500s and early 1600s, when the ancestors of some of us first set off across the Atlantic in search of a better life, scurvy and rickets were taking thousands of lives before the historic ships ever reached America's shores. Unprepared for the primitive life of the New World, women and babies died in childbirth, and nature's bitter elements took many lives as well. Native American healers, familiar with the restorative powers of their lands, shared shamanic teachings about the healing properties of plants, grains, and community. Recognizing the value of these natural remedies, the earliest settlers continued the medical evolution by sending these ideas back to Europe to incorporate them with the European healing tradition.

As the oceans' waters ebb and flow across sand, pebbles, and jagged rocks, so has medical theory over the centuries. The eclectic blend of Native American, African, Eastern, and European traditions eventually evolved into the new medicine: the Western way—the path that continues to dominate our medical treatments today. Corresponding with the U.S. industrial revolution, the mid-1800s marked an end to the free-spirited, anything-goes medicine of earlier times. Just like factory managers, physicians began to value the importance of fixing parts and keeping our bodies working like finely oiled machines. This type of thinking, along with the concept that bacteria produce disease and that antitoxins could be used to ward off these bacteria, formed the early roots of biomedicine. The American Medical Association was formed in 1847, and by the end of the nineteenth century its members were lobbying for state licensing laws. In the twentieth century, Western biomedical theory, as the conventional route to caring for the sick, was designated the one true path to health. Virtually every state in the United States passed laws governing medicine and its practice.

Because the medical establishment was quick to label alternative approaches to the Western way as hocus-pocus and quackery, chiropractors, homeopaths, and practitioners from other schools of thought (often women) were pushed out of the mainstream medical arena. The Pure Food and Drug Act, regulating the prescription of medicinals, was passed by 1906. With the release of the Flexner Report, *Medical Education in the United States and Canada,* in 1910, competing forms of medicine were virtually obliterated. Abraham Flexner, a U.S. educator and founder of the Institute for Advanced Study in Princeton, New Jersey, developed the report to set standards for American medical school education. In some instances the report helped regulate education, which in the 1800s had been far from adequate, ensuring that doctors were qualified to care for the ill and infirm.

But the Flexner Report certainly had its shortcomings: it was rigid, leaving little room for innovation and flexibility in medical education, and it never addressed the patient-doctor relationship. At the time that the Flexner Report was written, this relationship was taken for granted. Of course, the patient would always be considered above all else, Flexner reasoned. So he did not write that concept into the standards. As generations of doctors learned how to treat human bodies, that's all they learned. The importance of listening and staying connected to the patient was lost somewhere between anatomy and pharmacy. And even Flexner, who was not a physician, was eventually displeased with the rigid standards that he had originally helped create.

Within a few short years following Flexner's curricula guide, alternative medical schools—schools of homeopathy and osteopathy to name two—were left with little more than fringe status, and most were forced to close their doors. (Homeopathy is a school of treatment involving the administration of minute doses of remedies to increase the symptoms a patient is experiencing in an effort to spur the body's powers to restore harmony. Osteopathy is the science of manipulating the musculoskeletal system to restore health.) Biomedicine was the standard. Doctors and the powerful lobby of the AMA successfully kept the "charlatans," as they called them, out of the arena for nearly sixty years. It wasn't until consumer confidence in conventional medicine started to wane three decades ago that an opening appeared for alternative paths of healing. Many of the changes began to emerge in the sixties. Reports on the serious side effects of commonly used drugs like antibiotics started chipping away at consumer confidence. Coupled with a resurgence of more virulent strains of tuberculosis and deadly bacterial species like strep-A (the flesh-eater), not to mention new diseases like AIDS and Alzheimer's and cancer that traditional treatments could not cure, medical shoppers began looking for more. They wanted to find something to help them feel better, not necessarily get rid of the disease, just make them feel better. They wanted a more satisfying way of life.

MEDICINE AMERICAN-STYLE

Western Miracles and the Deification of Doctors

Many of this country's medical breakthroughs have had some basis in ancient Eastern wisdom. Drawing on an eleventh-century Chinese practice of using a powder derived from aging smallpox scabs to prevent disease, English country doctor Edward Jenner further evolved this Asian discovery into a vaccine for smallpox. Jenner scratched eight-year-old James Phipps's arm with the cowpox virus. It was this simple experiment that, several generations later, led to the eradication of smallpox in America and most of the world.[7] Although it was the Chinese who first used this technique, Jenner was named the Father of Vaccinology.

By the first half of this century, new medical discoveries had dramatically altered the face of Western medicine. Soaring past ancient horizons, medicine's innovations unveiled frontiers never before explored by even the most adventurous of healers. British bacteriologist Alexander Fleming was one such pathfinder. Returning from vacation in 1928, the pioneering scientist was cleaning up his laboratory and discarding used culture plates, when he observed something new: a fungus that had been flourishing on the culture plates in his absence was destroying the fringes of the deadly staphylococcus bacteria that had been smeared on the plates. His observations, although not fully appreciated and developed into penicillin until the 1940s, gave rise to a new era of treatment.[8]

At the same time government, academia, medical science, and the private sector, namely, drug companies with big dollars, formed previously unheard of alliances. Vast sums of government dollars were poured into medical research at medical schools and universities, and this powerful partnership[9] began a miraculous wave of invention that launched Western medical care into an age of wondrous findings and technological advances. Smallpox and polio were virtually eradicated in the Western hemisphere; human eggs could be fertilized in test tubes instead of in the mother's womb; surgery and medical imaging, enhanced by computers and robotics, became commonplace; body organs could be transplanted from dead patients into living ones, from pigs to humans; and through innovations in communication, and remote surgery techniques, surgeons and patients could remain on opposite sides of the country during surgical procedures.

As we approach the end of this millennium, technology is advancing more rapidly than even such sci-fi legends as Robert Heinlein or Isaac Asimov could predict. We're entering the twenty-first century with people living well into their eighties and nineties; forty- and fifty-year-old women (an age that once marked the end of life) are giving birth; aging, withered bodies are being sustained by transplants, respirators, and feeding tubes, while women and men voluntarily hook themselves up to the Kevorkian death machine when they can no longer tolerate the pain of living with debilitating diseases.

It's no wonder that we've been misguided into thinking that our doctors, our external healers, are deities capable of performing the greatest of miracles. We don't just pray for such miracles; we expect them. When a doctor fails to meet our ever increasing demands for youth and immortality, we sue. We scream malpractice. Doctors work in fear of litigation, often feeling it necessary to order a battery of unnecessary and expensive tests.[10]

An Era of Alienation

For the first time in history, we're a generation for the most part sadly lacking the wisdom of those who went before us. We've abdicated responsibility for our health and turned our health problems to teams of specialists. And these doctors, not being generalists, are not in a position to see us as whole human beings. The result is alienation of the doctor and the patient.

We seem to have lost touch with common sense, that inner knowing that tells us the baby's cold needs to run its course, or you should elevate your foot and stay off it if you've twisted your ankle—the doctor would say the same thing. There was a time when cultures relied on this most valuable resource, common sense.

We have lost sight of the fact that healing messages are as individual as the beings searching for a cure. Because of medical progress, it has become easier to view the human body as a machine: take a number, line up, cut it out, cut it off; get the broken or diseased part fixed; forget about it. We have become faceless body parts in the medical maze. Doctors admit that it's easy to forget there is a person attached to the gallbladder, the lung, the breast.

One surgeon shared a story with me. He had recently done a routine gallbladder surgery on an older woman. Returning to his office for the postoperative exam, she stood clutching her fine leather bag as he breezed in to check her progress. He started talking, asking her questions. He didn't recognize her, but that was a pretty common thing since he had gotten so busy. He didn't recognize lots of patients. But the woman had this puzzled look on her face. "Who are you?" she asked indignantly, stopping him dead. Momentarily he thought, "Who am I? I'm the surgeon." He realized that he had never examined this woman while she was conscious, and that through arrogance he assumed all his patients knew him; after all, he *was* the doctor. This was a defining moment for him, and he actually left his group practice shortly after this seemingly benign encounter. This woman, with the gallbladder, clutching her bag, brought this well-known surgeon to his knees.

Dare or Death: It's A Game of Life Roulette

Life Roulette. The stakes soar faster than the wheel can turn. As we throw down a growing stack of cash for one more try in the game, pieces of doctors and patients dissipate among the ashes of malpractice, managed care, dwindling resources, and the needless, violent deaths. Children. Old people. No one is spared the pain of a medical system crying out for change. Perhaps it's the dwindling financial and human resources, or the mutant bacterial strains that antibiotics will no longer heal. Or is it cancer? AIDS? Violence? Guns? Gangs? Our inner city emergency rooms are turning thousands of patients away. Lined-up in halls, in waiting rooms, on park benches, their plea becomes a whisper lost in the murky residue of noise, cars, sirens and too many others. Quiet moments at any emergency room are rare, and they come suddenly, like the yellow-green stillness that falls over the trees, streets, and trailers just before the tornado's black funnel sweeps victims in its wake. While some patients are fortunate enough to have family or insurance to care for their needs, others are forced to seek solace in shelters rather than in the arms of a loved one. Others die, unnoticed, under bridges, near trash cans, in back alleys, in their cardboard beds.

Are We Managing Care, or Is It Managing Us?

Every one of us suffers for the needless excesses of our health care system. When most of our grandfathers, fathers, sons, or lovers were across the ocean fighting in World War II and women were working in factories, national health care dollars spent were about $4 billion. Half a century later, in 1992, the money spent on health care each year had soared to $800 billion, and conservative estimates indicate that number will soon exceed a trillion dollars.[11]

Back in 1940, most health care costs for doctors and hospitals went to cover the most serious, acute conditions. Today the situation seems to have flipped: the seriously ill are forced home in two or three days, no longer able to get well in a hospital setting. These are stays that in the past were treated in hospital settings for eight to ten days. Now, thanks to the health insurance industry, major surgical procedures for things such as mastectomies warrant a twenty-four-hour stay, while treatments for chronic conditions such as arthritis, pain, depression, and high blood pressure eat up about 70 percent of the current health care budget. According to the U.S. Department of Health and Human Services publication *Healthy People 2000,* more than 33 million Americans are functionally restricted from daily activities because of such chronic conditions.

Managed care has become our solution to the rising costs of health care. But insurers further muddy the waters by insisting that our care be dictated by the dollar and the day. Too many days, too much money equals time to go home. You're still sick, you say? The ever-tightening noose of managed care and its capitation system have become part of medical treatment delivery, while patients, doctors, families, government leaders—everyone—is asking, *why?* We are told that because as a nation we shell out $950 billion annually to care for our sick, we need to find ways to cut costs, so that everyone can be served. We can no longer afford to pay for everyone to be treated for every ailment.

We are the only industrialized nation with no comprehensive system of health care delivery. More than 37 million Americans have no health insurance, and 22 million working poor go untreated because they cannot afford adequate coverage. Others, with the right amount of money, the right job, and the best insurance, continue to enjoy the luxury of being covered for elective procedures. The health care controversy even took over the 1992 presidential campaign, placing First Lady Hillary Rodham Clinton under a microscope of public scrutiny. There were focus groups. There was testimony. There was posturing and grandstanding. And everybody was trying to get on the list of speakers: the special interests, the hospital administrators, the business leaders, the doctors, the patients, the insurers. Everybody had to have his or her story heard. But try as the First Lady might, she could not make the pieces of the puzzle fit. And now that the dust has settled after the whirlwind of a failed attempt, it's clear that no winners emerged from this damaging battle. Some favored a national health care plan. Some were vehemently opposed. Some only cared about protecting their niche in the health care arena. The patients— and when you think about it, we're all patients at some point— wanted affordable, accessible, quality care. To make matters worse, the golden crescent of scientific evidence that's all wrapped up in the double-blind bind of clinical trials and proof, kept raising its ugly head, as a few brave souls tried to consider alternative options to conventional care. And now, several years later, we're still puzzled. We ask, How did this happen? What role did we play? Many are quick to blame the other guy: the hospitals; the doctors; the insurance companies; the uninsured; the government; the gangs; the guns; the immigrants; the homosexuals. No matter who gets saddled with the blame, the questions remain: Who will pay? Who will get care, and who will die without it?

The answer may not be the cure. Perhaps the simple truth of healing is connecting or reconnecting to the inner healer within each of us. Maybe it's learning to live with grace and ease, with or without cancer, AIDS, or addiction. Or could it be that we have to unleash the power of centuries of knowledge, taking a little wisdom and a little loving and mixing it up with a lot of common sense? Many doctors today think that we have lost touch with our generational wisdom. Generations before us knew the answer. They had a special tea for this and an herb or poultice for that. Only when things seemed fairly grim was the doctor summoned. Some feel that doctors didn't always know the answers anyway. And that was OK. They, too, relied on an invisible force for the answers. But today, the practice of Western medicine has far surpassed such folksy remedies. It took the doctor out of the village and threw this once familiar healer into the vast hive of buzzing competition and technology. Our grandmothers easily diagnosed the difference between croup and pneumonia. But the post- World War II era tossed common sense out the window. And we lost a sense of generational wisdom. We invalidated the lessons of generations before us. Old people were old, not smart. We were young, hip, and strong. Times were good. We had jobs, money, and education. We had color television, and the world got smaller as technology progressed. Our families split: a brother "in California; his wife and children in Indiana; a sister in Florida; parents up North. We kept moving so fast that no one from the class reunion committee would ever be able to find us again. We were lost in the blur of express living and fun times. And now we're all alone.

A MEETING OF THE MINDS:
A NEW APPROACH TO HEALING

For thousands of years, healers have been trying to uncover the ever changing mysteries of the human body. Both the Eastern and Western traditions go back many centuries. The Eastern tradition is steeped in philosophy and spirituality, and, in its approach to healing, the body is seen as a microcosm of nature, a landscape of the seen and the unseen, whose seasons and temperatures, deficiencies and excesses need to be gauged and understood in order to promote health. At one time the Western tradition had some similar beliefs, the Greeks, for example, seeing disease as an imbalance in the four humors, but since the 1800s, a lot of that tradition has been overshadowed by the Cartesian thinking of modern medicine, which views the body as a machine, a mechanical structure that can be diagnosed based on cause-and-effect thinking, and whose parts can be removed and replaced or molded or zapped into shape; and which views disease as a separate entity with its own patterns and cycles that are to be disrupted and put out of commission through drugs or surgery. The healing wisdom of centuries in the West was overshadowed by this approach to medicine. But practitioners and patients are now regaining a sense that the systems and organs of the human body are interdependent parts of an organic whole, and that curing what ails us involves encouraging the body to fight for wholeness rather than target and destroy symptoms. Medicine is so intriguing today because the West is continuing to learn more about cells, immunity, disease, and genetics, while it eagerly explores Eastern medicine, tapping into the wealth of wisdom it offers. The prospect of our getting the benefit of all these systems, practices, and wisdom bodes well for our general health and well-being.

Medicine's emerging heroes—Bernie Siegel, Andrew Weil, Larry Dossey, Deepak Chopra, Dean Ornish, Christiane Northrup, and Sandra McLanahan, to name a few—have, through experimentation, new findings, and ancient teachings extracted the prime nectar of all the available medical worlds. The pilgrimage to integrative medicine, to wellness, has just begun.

> "There are some very good things about Western medicine, but many times it is used to treat patients across the board. Everybody gets the same treatment. Healing depends on the person, and everyone needs custom-designed health care. I let patients talk for the first hour or so, so they can unload and get it all out. They talk, they cry, and

from that point on I go into my complete physical, which combines Eastern and Western diagnostic tools. Using Eastern principles in treatment is not some fly-by-night, silly little therapy. It's not New Agey; it's Old Agey. It's been around for more than 2,500 years."

—Carolyn Jaffe, nationally certified acupuncturist, registered with the Pennsylvania State Department of Osteopathic Medicine, Diplomat of acupuncture

The birth of integrative medicine will force the medical establishment to form previously unheard of alliances with practitioners once shunned by Western medicine. Transforming the course of our nation's curative path, our sick care system will become obsolete. New strategies, blending the spiritual, emotional, and natural with high-tech procedures, will evolve. Although it may seem overwhelming, this change is close at hand.

OUR HEALTH CARE SYSTEM IS NOT EMULATED THROUGHOUT THE WORLD

People in the U.S. think of Western medicine as the standard method of care, often assuming that the rest of the world practices medicine as we do. In actuality, estimates reveal that only 10 to 30 percent of the world's health care is delivered by conventional Western methods; the remaining 70 to 90 percent is rendered by alternative modes of treatment.[12]

THE BIRTH OF INTEGRATIVE MEDICINE: GESTATION, TWENTY-SEVEN YEARS

"Most of the people who come to me are ready for something different because they have tried what doesn't work. We don't have a health care system; we have an illness system. One thing integrative medicine can do is teach people. And that will begin to provide the tools for change."
—Sandra McLanahan, M.D., executive medical director of the Integral Health Center in Buckingham, Virginia, and physician to the world-renowned spiritual healer Reverend Sri Swami Satchidananda

1971 *New York Times* columnist James Reston brings the concept of acupuncture and Chinese herbs to America's shores.

1983 The Alternative Health Plan is established in California by Steve and Sherry Gorman. The company's goal is to provide medical plans offering freedom of choice and including coverage for alternative and complementary medicine such as acupuncture, massage, and herbal remedies.

1986 The Oriental Medical Center in Los Angeles studies the efficacy of Chinese herbs and acupuncture in treating ARC and AIDS.

1992 The nation's first federally funded alternative medicine HIV public health clinic project gets underway in San Francisco.

The Office of Alternative Medicine, part of the National Institutes of Health, is created by Congress. This is the first federal agency focusing on alternative treatments.

1993 Harvard University researcher Dr. David Eisenberg releases findings in the *New England Journal of Medicine* on Americans' use of alternative therapies. This landmark study reports that one in three Americans used at least one form of unconventional therapy.

American Western Life Insurance Company offers its first wellness plan, which promotes self-care and reimbursements for visits to alternative practitioners.

1994 A Gallup poll finds that 17 percent of Americans use herbal supplements, a 14 percent increase over the previous year.

The Dietary Supplement Health and Education Act is passed by Congress, deregulating herbal remedies.

The first two specialty research centers—Bastyr University AIDS Research Center, Seattle, and Minneapolis Medical Research Center for Addictions Study—are established by the NIH to study the effects of alternative therapies.

Health insurance giant Blue Cross and Blue Shield of Washington and Alaska launches a year long pilot program, Alterna Path, which provides coverage for alternative treatments.

1995 Kaiser Permanente, the country's largest health maintenance organization, opens the doors of its first alternative medicine clinic in Vallejo, California.

Harvard Medical School hosts the first-of-its-kind mind/body conference for doctors, who can receive continuing education credits for attending.

Eight specialty research centers have now joined the NIH Office of Alternative Medicine in its efforts to study alternative medicine.

The State of Washington passes a law requiring all insurance companies to cover the services of licensed alternative practitioners.

1996 The State of Oregon follows Washington's lead and presents voters with the Healthcare Freedom Initiative, a plan similar to that of Washington State, but it fails at the polls because of a technicality.

The first-of-its-kind nationwide study of patient perceptions of Chinese medicine treatments is conducted under the direction of the Traditional Acupuncture Institute in Columbia, Maryland.

The first clinical study of the effects of the Chinese herb dong quai on postmenopausal women is conducted by Kaiser Permanente's Division of Research. A record number of volunteers express interest in participating.

Acupuncture needles are removed from the FDA's list of investigational devices, making them accepted treatment devices, no longer considered experimental.

One of the first undergraduate courses in unconventional medicine is offered at the University of California, Davis.

The Asian Diet Pyramid is released.

1997 National Institutes of Health Office of Alternative Medicine and the Office of Dietary Supplements are collaborating to fund research on the benefits of the herb commonly known as St. John's Wort as a potential treatment for depression.

National Institutes of Health panel endorses acupuncture therapy as an effective treatment for certain types of pain, nausea, as a surgical anesthesia, for pregnancy, and to relieve the side effects of chemotherapy. The panel also says that there is evidence that acupuncture may be effective for menstrual cramps, tennis elbow, drug addiction, stroke, and fibromyalgia.

Teaching Alternative Treatments at Traditional Medical Schools

Eastern applications and Western alternatives have been quietly creeping into the mainstream Western medical practices. Hospitals around the country now offer some form of alternative (the term used to define anything unproven in Western medical terms) choice for patients. Western medical schools are adding integrative medicine courses, for example, blending Chinese medicine with Western therapies, to their once conservative curricula. Therapies until recently considered offbeat and unproven—such as acupuncture, meditation, herbology, energy balancing, spirituality, and various cultural traditions—now complement traditional training. Conservative Columbia University has created the Richard and Hinda Rosenthal Center for Alternative/Complementary Medicine. Harvard Medical School offers students an intensive course on alternative medical practices.

According to information from the Office of Alternative Medicine at the National Institutes of Health, there are more than twenty-six prominent medical schools now offering courses in alternative medicine. Yale School of Medicine, Temple University, Johns Hopkins School of Medicine, Stanford University School of Medicine, Mount Sinai School of Medicine, Harvard Medical School, Columbia University College of Physicians, Emory University School of Medicine, and the University of Virginia Medical School are among them.

FELLOWSHIP PROGRAM AT THE UNIVERSITY OF ARIZONA

The University of Arizona College of Medicine developed the nation's first postgraduate fellowship program in integrative medicine. Under the direction of best-selling author Dr. Andrew Weil, the Arizona program accepts board-certified physicians to a course of study that includes acupuncture, herbology, visualization, mind/body techniques, Chinese medicine, and Native American medicine, to name a few. According to materials developed for the program, it was created in response to a growing demand from physicians for instruction in alternative healing practices.

"It is anticipated that this pioneer program in integrative medicine will help document which of the alternative medical approaches to include in standard allopathic practice. . . .

I am personally convinced that many of the interventions studied and used in this innovative program will find their way into future daily allopathic practice. At that time, the term alternative will no longer be appropriate for these techniques and agents. Indeed they will have become mainstream therapy."[13]

—Joseph S. Alpert, M.D., head of the Department of Medicine, Arizona Health Sciences Center, University of Arizona College of Medicine

Goals of the University of Arizona Program in Integrative Medicine

- To train doctors to combine the best ideas and practices of conventional and alternative medicine into new cost-effective treatments.
- To encourage doctors to research theories and methods of alternative systems of treatment.
- To encourage doctors to be role models of healthy living.
- To provide integrative medical care for a selected group of patients coming to the university health center.
- To develop a model of training that can be used by other medical institutions.
- To produce leaders for this new discipline of medicine who will establish similar programs at other institutions and set policy and direction for health care in the twenty-first century.[14]

HEALING OPTIONS COURSE AT
UNIVERSITY OF VIRGINIA MEDICAL SCHOOL

About seven years ago a group of medical students approached Pali DeLevitt, Ph.D., saying they needed her to teach a course at the medical school. A cancer survivor who had found healing through her own disease and the use of alternative methods, DeLevitt was known for her strong spirituality and her understanding of the healing process. Teaching a course at the medical school wasn't exactly what she saw in her future, but after giving it some thought she developed a curriculum and approached the head of the medical school with her concepts for an alternative healing course. DeLevitt recalls that there was surprisingly little resistance to what she was proposing, so she began teaching what has become an extremely popular elective for fourth-year medical students.

At a healing space she has created in the woods just behind her Charlottesville, Virginia, home, DeLevitt introduces students to drug and surgical alternative options for treating patients and spends a great deal of time helping them get in touch with their own healing and spirituality. As part of the intensive monthlong course, the medical students are required to participate in group meditation as well as commit to make lifestyle changes at least for the duration of the course. They go out in the field and learn from alternative practitioners, where they discover that there are nonharmful herbal remedies that in some instances can take the place of most prescription drugs; that acupuncture, massage, and energy healing can be very effective in relieving pain; and that the relationship between the doctor and patient needs to be very intimate. She says that the students are amazed, often asking, "How come in four years of medical school no one told us about these things?"

"Medical school students get indoctrinated into drug and surgical management," she says. "But rarely do they hear about healing; everything is disease symptom oriented."

Because she requires that students take a Western diagnosis and research how that particular ailment might be treated with alternative methods, the students leave the course knowing that there are treatment options for various disorders. "If a patient comes to you with asthma, it is your role to inform them that they have alternatives to drug therapy," she tells the students. She told me, "These medical students are the vanguard of new healers. A doctor should be able to look at the many possibilities of the human experience and be able to discuss these things with their patients."

> *"This course changed my life. I will never look at things the same way again. It not only changed the way I will practice medicine; it changed the way I will live."*
>
> —a fourth-year University of Virginia medical student referring to DeLevitt's alternative medicine course, Healing Options, offered at the medical school

The National Institutes of Health Joins the Act

What some have called unorthodox therapies are gaining even more credibility, or at least a second look, even from the harshest critics.

The creation of the National Institutes of Health's (NIH) Office of Alternative Medicine (OAM) has spurred this growth. In 1996 the OAM, under the direction of Wayne Jonas, M.D., a family physician with a background in many alternative therapies including homeopathy, bioenergy, and spiritual healing, awarded nearly $9.7 million in grants to ten institutions to conduct research on the therapeutic merits of Chinese herbs, acupuncture, massage, and other alternatives to conventional Western medical treatment. In a hearing before the Senate Labor and Human Resources Committee regarding the Access to Medical Treatment Act, Jonas testified that the OAM is committed to accelerating public access to potentially useful complementary and alternative therapies.

The OAM's leader reports that his office is exploring methods to assess and monitor the results of individual practices of complementary and alternative health practitioners, including practice-based research networks. Jonas has recommended a three-tiered review process specifically tailored to judge the level of risk of particular treatments. He states, "If such developments were accompanied by systematic data collection of selected unapproved therapies, a situation allowing access, assuring public safety, and furthering research could be accomplished."[15]

The following is a list of NIH Office of Alternative Medicine initial grant awards. Although research in these directions is improving, it is clear how comparatively little is spent on research in alternative therapies.

Dartmouth-Hitchcock Medical Center $29,901
Massage Therapy for Bone Marrow Transplant

University of Arizona $29,585
Acupuncture, Unipolar Depression

University of Maryland Pain Center $30,000
Acupuncture, Osteoarthritis

Medical College of Ohio $26,405
Massage Therapy, HIV-1

City of Hope National Medical Center $30,000
Electrochemical DC Current, Cancer

American Health Foundation $30,000
Pancreatic Enzyme Therapy, Cancer

Virginia Polytechnic Institute and State University $30,000
Hypnosis, Low Back Pain

University of Virginia School of Medicine $28,919
Massage Therapy, Post-Surgical Outcomes

Pacific College of Oriental Medicine $30,000
Chinese Herbal Medicine, PMS

Washington University $30,000
Anti-Hepatitis Plants, Therapeutic Evaluation

Pennsylvania State University $30,000
Music Therapy, Psychosocial Adjustment after Brain Injury

Menninger Clinic $30,000
Energetic Therapy Basal Cell Carcinoma

University of Miami School of Medicine $30,000
Massage Therapy, HIV-Exposed Infants

Harvard Medical School $30,000
Hypnosis, Accelerated Bone Fracture Healing

University of California $30,000
Classical Homeopathy, Health Status

Hahnemann University, $18,420
Dance/Movement Therapy, Cystic Fibrosis

Emory University $30,000
Chinese Herbal Therapy, Common Warts

George Washington University $29,985
Imagery and Relaxation, Immunity Control

Northwestern University $29,985
T'ai-Chi, Mild Balance Disorders

Lenox Hill Hospital $30,000
Guided Imagery, Asthma

University of Texas Health Science Center $30,000
Imagery and Relaxation, Breast Cancer

University of Vermont $30,000
Manual Palpation, Lumbar Spine

Columbia University $30,000
Chinese Herbs, Hot Flashes

University of Minnesota $29,964
Macrobiotic Diet, Cancer

Alternative Treatments Gaining Popularity among Doctors and Consumers

Alternative therapy is fast becoming a $15 billion industry in this country. And many of the nearly 670,000 Western conventional, or allopathic, medical doctors in this nation have demonstrated an increasing openness to the possibility that alternative therapies may have merit. The first original published research, led by David Blumberg, M.D., of the department of psychiatry at the State University of New York Health Science Center at Syracuse, reported that over 90 percent of the doctors responding to survey questions said that they were willing to refer their patients for an alternative form of treatment. These findings were based on 572 responses to 2,000 questionnaires that were mailed to conventionally trained and board-certified internists and family physicians.

In late 1995, the results of a study published in the *Archives of Internal Medicine* stated that "on average physicians perceive complementary medicine as moderately effective, with younger physicians more receptive than their older counterparts." Nonetheless, the study concluded by saying that these alternative therapies " urgently need to be tested in randomized controlled trials." Proponents of alternative therapies say that such testing won't work because of the unquantifiable components of many alternative therapies, including spirituality, energy, human interaction, and placebo effects. And in symposia and medical conferences around the nation during 1996, that point continued to be debated among the nation's top healers.

"It's an enormous problem. They are stalled around the methodological issue, how do you research this? And right now the methodological issues are virtually insurmountable. I think they're missing the point. They are always looking for the control group. Researching common sense gets very expensive."

—Robert Duggan, president of the Traditional
Acupuncture Institute, Columbia, Maryland, and former chair of the Maryland State Board of Acupuncture

Back in 1993 David Eisenberg, M.D., and a group of researchers from Harvard reported in the *New England Journal of Medicine* on their findings from a telephone survey of 1,539 respondents. The team discovered that in 1990 one in three American adults relied on an unconventional treatment for a health problem. Unconventional, for this study, was defined as meaning medical interventions not taught widely at U.S. medical schools or available at U.S. hospitals. The study also reported that Americans had made more visits to alternative practitioners—425 million—than to primary care doctors— 388 million—during that year. Amazingly, these same adults shelled out more than $13.7 billion for unconventional care, three-fourths of which came from their own pockets.

This past year, a Harvard-based study of medical directors of Health Maintenance Organizations (HMOs) in thirteen states found that chiropractic and acupuncture are the top two alternative therapies that HMOs plan to offer their members within the next one to two years.

Here are some other survey highlights:

- 58 percent of the respondents indicated that they plan to offer alternative care therapies to members in the next two years;
- 70 percent reported an increase in requests for alternative care therapies from members;
- acupuncture, massage, and chiropractic were the top three therapies of interest to HMO members.

OTHER TRENDS IN ALTERNATIVE MEDICINE

- Insurers are loosening the noose around the necks of alter-native practitioners, and one of the first to change was the once conservative Blue Cross of Washington and Alaska.

After conducting a series of town meetings across the state, Blue Cross launched AlternaPath, a pilot program covering naturopathy, homeopathy, and acupuncture. Enrollees paid $171 for up to $1,000 of treatment, and the pilot was limited to 1,000 subscribers. The program was filled to capacity within three months.

- American Western Life of Foster City, California is another insurance company at the forefront with regard to alternative medicine. The company's wellness plan, available to individuals in Arizona, California, New Mexico, and Colorado, is one of the first to offer coverage for alternative and traditional treatments.
- State of Washington lawmakers passed legislation that mandated that all insurers and managed care organizations make the coverage of services for licensed alternative health care providers available to subscribers. Taking effect in January 1996, the ground-breaking Washington law set the stage for an Oregon proposal, the Healthcare Freedom Initiative, which failed on a technicality in the November 1996 elections.
- Oxford Health Plans, a managed care company based in Norwalk, Connecticut, announced plans in late 1996 to become the first large medical insurer to offer a network of alternative care providers. Starting in early 1997, the Oxford Health options became available to individuals and employers in Connecticut, New Jersey, Pennsylvania, and New York. For employers adding the alternative option to their benefits packages, premiums will increase by about $5 to $6 a member per year.
- A hotline for health care practitioners—Natural Healthcare Hotline, a service developed by the Natural Healthcare Institute—has been established to provide access to research-based information on alternative health care products.

NATION'S FIRST PUBLICLY FUNDED NATURAL MEDICINE CLINIC: COMMUNITY HEALTH CENTERS OF KING COUNTY AND BASTYR

The Community Health Centers, a national nonprofit agency that provides care for underserved populations, will house one of the nation's first publicly funded natural medicine clinics in its Kent, Washington, center. In conjunction with Bastyr University and the Statistics and Epidemiology Research Corporation, Community Health Centers plans to offer natural medicine treatment to low-income, immigrant, and refugee populations in the Seattle area.

Natural medicine involves restoring health through encouraging the elimination of toxins. Practitioners of naturopathy believe that health is maintained by avoiding unnatural or artificial products in the environment and diet. Poor lifestyle habits are often corrected through adopting new behaviors in terms of eating, exercising, attitude, and self-care.

Alternative therapies will be available to these populations in addition to conventional treatment already available at the center. The clinic has $750,000 in funding, approved by the Washington State Legislature, which is provided by a State Legalization and Immigration Assistance grant. The research corporation will conduct studies evaluating patient satisfaction, cost-effectiveness, and health outcomes, and these findings will be compared to results for conventional therapies for the following health conditions: migraine headaches, high blood pressure, chronic ear infections, and asthma. Bastyr, an accredited natural medicine school and an OAM-funded specialty research center investigating alternative therapies for HIV/AIDS, will manage the clinic.

OUR LEGACY

The medical revolution is at hand. And perhaps the most active rebels will be you and me, those of us looking for a better way to wellness. As we evaluate our own desires, examine our beliefs, we will uncover the healing powers stored within our bodies. Many—from all over the globe—will walk beside us on this journey. Even Western practitioners, who once thought that the Western way was the *only* way, will join us as we discover an elegant route to wellness—a route that integrates the natural, the spiritual, the personal, with the technological advances of our modern world. Through integrative medicine, we begin our journey together. This is the legacy we will leave for future generations.

"I had been feeling unhappy. I was offered a trial of Prozac by my medical doctor. I compared the cost of Prozac (100% out-of-pocket) and that of psychotherapy and acupuncture (receiving 40% and 75% reimbursement respectively) and though it's about half the cost to use Prozac, I decided I wanted human contact and an opportunity to be coached and educated into how to grasp my struggles in life better. Also, I quit my job . . . for one that is much less stressful. I feel less depressed and a whole lot smarter. I care about the people I work with, too."

—Male, 21–30 age group, survey respondent

WESTERN MEDICINE'S FIRSTS

1796 Edward Jenner first inoculates against smallpox.

1847 The American Medical Association is formed.

1892 The American Medicinal Plants is compiled. It is the first American-based herbal medicinal, containing information on the healing properties of 180 plants.

1928 The first antibiotic is discovered by Alexander Fleming.

1938 The first cardiac catheterization is performed in New York by George Peter Robb and Israel Steinberg.

1953 DNA's double-helix structure is discovered by Francis Crick and James Watson.

1955 There is a major public health effort to inoculate children with the polio vaccine discovered by Jonas Salk.

1957 Oral polio vaccine is formulated by Jonas Salk.

1957 Fiber optic endoscopy is pioneered by Basil Hirschowtiz at the University of Michigan.

1967 The first human heart transplant is carried out by Christiaan Barnard.

1972 Computed tomography, CAT scans, are devised by British engineers.

1978 First test-tube baby is born in England.

1979 The World Health Organization declares that smallpox has been eradicated.

1981 The Centers for Disease Control is alerted to the first reported cases of AIDS, occurring in Los Angeles and New York.

1981 The MRI scanner is developed by scientists at Nottingham University and Thorn-EMI Laboratories in England.

1985 The first PET scanner is developed by researchers at the University of California, a technique that enables organ functioning to be studied in color.

EASTERN MEDICINE'S FIRSTS

2700 B.C. The legendary emperor Shen-nung is credited with writing the first recorded history of medicinal herbs and plants. This pharmacopoeia has been called the *PenTsao*. As legend has it, Shen-nung tasted all the herbs to test their value and use. He lived for 123 years.

2600 B.C. The first written presentation of comprehensive medical theory is produced, *The Nei Ching Su Wen* or *The Yellow Emperor's Classic of Internal Medicine*.

300 B.C. The first anesthetic powder is developed for surgical procedures such as laparotomies and wound expansions by Hua Tuo, Chinese physician.

1066–225 B.C. Environmental hygiene, personal hygiene, boiling water, and the elimination of rats and rabid dogs to prevent disease are espoused by Zhou dynasty, China.

1000–221 B.C. The first integrated system of medicinal classification (for herbs) is created in China.

320 A.D. The first study of pharmaceutical chemistry is developed by Ge Hong, a Chinese physician in the Jin dynasty.

Eleventh Century People are inoculated with the serum of human smallpox in China.

618–1279 Medicine is divided into branches in China relating to the treatment of diseases and bodily functions—orthopedics, laryngology, wounds, acupuncture, gynecology, ophthalmology, and stomatology.

1247 The first book of forensic medicine is written by Song Ci in China.

1949 After the 1949 revolution, the People's Republic of China brings Chinese medicine back into prominence, establishing organized training for practitioners.

1971 *New York Times* reporter James Reston is taken to Chinese hospital for emergency appendectomy. He later writes of the benefits of acupuncture and Chinese herbal medicine.

1976 Chinese gynecologists develop chorionic villus sampling, an aid to early diagnosis of genetic disorders.

Blending East and West: Searching for Your Garden

"Taoists see man as a microcosm of the universe and the body as a reflection of one's attunement of the cycles, rhythms, and patterns of the larger universe."

—Tricia Yu, The T'ai-Chi Center, Madison, Wisconsin

Our bodies, much like gardens, need love, nourishment, tending, and rest, to flourish. We flow through the seasons year after year, winter to spring, summer to autumn, rarely giving thought to the natural course of things. The balance of the heavens, clouds, mountains, rains, and rivers are all part of nature's giving and taking, coming and going; much like the flow of blood, energy, and cell regeneration in our bodies. Our physical bodies, just as our lives, cycle through their own seasons. And with each new season comes a little dying, resting, rebirth, and growth. As a child, did you ever skin your knee and watch in wonder as the wound magically went through its healing cycle? Even more amazing was the seed that pushed its way through the moistened earth and turned into a tomato, or the tadpole that turned into a frog. It's all part of living, growing, and tending in nature's time and cycles. Rivers overflow their banks, sun bakes the ground dry, locusts or gypsy moths destroy the rich green leaves that form the brilliance of the tree's sturdy frame. In the natural world, disasters throw things out of balance, just like cancer, arthritis, or pneumonia can wreak havoc on our bodies. Did you ever notice how nature begins healing? It's much like when as children we watched in amazement as our skinned knee repaired itself. Healing is part of nature's design, and, although outside help sometimes moves the healing along, nature finds a way of regenerating life. Our bodies are much like this. It is our own inner ability to heal that does all the work, and we should look on practitioners, whether Eastern, Western, or a blended combination, as guides along the path, whether we are getting things back in balance so healing can take place, trying to improve our lifestyle, ridding our bodies of toxins, or resparking our internal energy. In the end, no matter what the approach, it is our individual healing ability that does the repair, the re-creating, and the healing.

THE EASTERN MODEL: YOUR BODY AS A LANDSCAPE

Twelve beautiful rivers flow along distinct meridians in the human body. Nourished by sun, wind, rain, earth, and fire, the seasons unfold as your lush internal landscape transforms with your seasonal changes. A cosmos of the two energies, yin and yang, dance the divine dance of night and day, heat and cold. And whether Traditional Chinese medicine, Five Element Chinese medicine, or Ayurveda, the healing of the body requires the rebalancing of the life force, taking into account a person's entire life—body, mind, and spirit.

The practice of traditional Oriental medicine is based on a highly sophisticated and complicated model of health care that has roots in the metaphysical worlds of Taoism, Buddhism, and Confucianism. Having spread throughout East Asia more than 2,500 years ago, this philosophy of healing considers the whole person and his or her relationship to the universe and all living and spiritual things. Although Oriental medicine is grounded in Chinese culture, there are variations in methods and therapies throughout Asian countries. Many of these most ancient approaches to health—acupuncture, herbalism, acupressure, *qigong*, and Oriental massage—are widely used throughout the world today. Many of the world's healing practices borrow or refine on the traditions of Oriental practitioners.

By the beginning of the Han dynasty, Oriental medicine was already a well-documented and practiced form of medical care. As the Han era ended, Chinese medicine was promoting prevention, diet, and the concept that medical practices should be judged by patient results. Chinese thought and practice continued to evolve through the Middle Ages and Western Europe's Renaissance, but during the colonial times, contact with Westerners pushed Oriental medicine into folk and religious realms. And it wasn't until the Communist regime of the People's Republic of China gave Oriental medicine credence that Chinese medicine experienced a resurgence and renewed growth. Since 1949 medical training, research, and advances in Oriental medicine have been great.

There are currently about 6,500 acupuncture practitioners and 1,600 practitioners of Chinese herbal medicine and Chinese massage in the United States. As acceptance of these modes of treatment grows, so does the number of practitioners. At this time, licensing varies by state; New Mexico is the most progressive, in that acupuncturists have a legal scope to practice that is similar to that of a primary care physician.

THE CONVENTIONAL WESTERN MODEL: YOUR BODY AS A FINELY TUNED MACHINE

The eclectic blend of Native American, African, Eastern, and European traditions, all of which claimed a piece of this country's soil in colonial and postcolonial America, eventually were all but replaced by Western biomedicine, which continues to dominate our health care options today. Although Hippocrates saw medicine as involving the whole person—including diet, lifestyle, and environment—the discovery of microorganisms such as bacteria and fungi led to the germ theory of disease which changed the way doctors looked at diagnosis. By the time of the American Industrial Revolution, Western doctors had developed new theories about the body and ways to repair it. Other medical traditions and modes were marginalized. Western medicine has evolved into a mechanistic discipline made up of doctors specializing in one bodily system or another and concentrating on using machines and drugs to treat symptoms, rather than seeing the disease as an imbalance in the whole organism. Just like factory managers, physicians began to value the importance of fixing parts and keeping our bodies working like finely oiled machines. From the late nineteenth century, biomedicine evolved quickly.

Principles of Chinese Medicine

THE SIX EVIL QI, THE SEVEN PASSIONS, AND THE FIVE ELEMENTS

Chinese medicine divides the causes of disease into categories, and, depending on the type of Chinese medicine practiced, there will be variations in the degree to which practitioners will stand behind some of these theories. Consisting of such therapies as acupuncture, moxibustion, cupping, therapeutic exercises, massage, and diet and lifestyle changes, Chinese medicine is based on the principle of balance and harmony. Some believe that when the six qi—wind, cold, summer, heat, dampness, dryness, and heat—are healthy, they reflect the natural progressions and fluctuations of our life as we travel through the seasons of the year. These six qi are all part of the natural balance of yin and yang. Only when they get out of balance, too much or too little, are they called the six evil qi. According to Chinese belief, sudden changes in the weather, our emotions, or our lifestyle can cause these qi to become blocked or imbalanced. Acupuncture and massage are ways to restore balance. The Chinese also believe that emotional factors—joy, anger, brooding, sadness, and fear—can cause disease, so they warn of avoiding excess passion. Many Chinese practitioners, those who practice Five-Element Chinese medicine in particular, also believe in the five elements of wood, fire, earth, metal, and water. According to Daniel Reid, the author of *The Complete Book of Chinese Health and Healing*, the five elements, unlike the Western system,

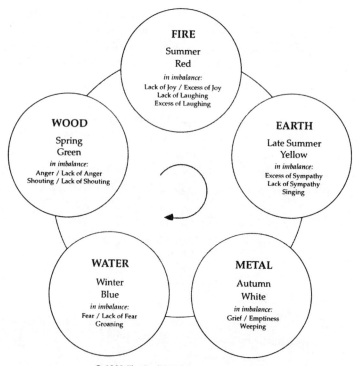

© 1992 The Traditional Acupuncture Institute

THE FIVE ELEMENTS

focus on energy and its transformations, not on form and substance. The elements thus symbolize the activities of the energies with which they are associated.[1] If one element predominates, the others will become unbalanced, and disease may occur. These elements give us the ability and the framework to be more connected in our daily life. And each of these elements represents certain colors, seasons, and emotions. Ancient Chinese healers understood the five elements by watching nature; they understood wood by watching trees growing; fire and heat by observing the sun; water quenched their thirst and put out fire; and so they began to understand their own healing process.

> *"In order to bring into harmony the human body one takes as standard the laws of the four seasons and the five elements."*
> —*The Nei Ching Su Wen,* or *The Yellow Emperor's Classic of Internal Medicine*

> *"The Chinese are poetic in their descriptions and diagnosis. For someone to get a good night's sleep, the* shen *(spirit) has to be anchored in the heart. When it is unanchored the heart can become too hot and dreams may disturb sleep. So if someone had a shen disturbance, we would treat the heart channel."*
> —Jody Forman, licensed acupuncturist

Eastern Diagnosis

LOOKING, LISTENING, ASKING, AND FEELING

Diagnosis in Oriental medicine involves the classical procedures of observation, listening, questioning, smelling, and feeling. From the moment an Eastern practitioner sets eyes on the patient—observing the gait, mannerisms, the hues and colors radiating off the face in natural light, the body type—the diagnostic process begins. Depending on whether the physician is guided by Traditional Chinese Medicine (TCM), Five-Element acupuncture, or Ayurveda, certain clues read from the patient aid the practitioner in making a diagnosis. It's rare that a skilled practitioner will miss these clues. For patients, this thorough going-over can be a little disconcerting on the first visit. But as Paul Olko, a practitioner of Chinese herbal medicine told me, he never makes personal judgments when diagnosing a patient. The longer a practitioner has been practicing his or her art, the more readily will the signs become part of the total assessment of the patient. By observing patient interviews and diagnosis I learned that most patients are starving for individualized attention to their body and their needs, so they appreciate the time and care Eastern practitioners take in assessing their needs.

A simple handshake can reveal much about the patient to the practitioner. He or she takes note of the texture, temperature, and moisture of the skin. Is the patient hot or cool? Damp or dry? Rough or smooth? How does the patient smell? How is the patient breathing? Is the patient's voice low or loud?

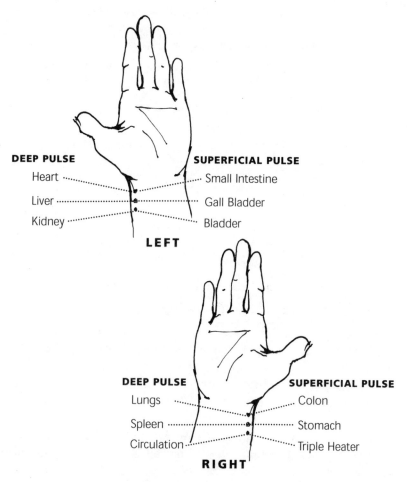

DEEP PULSE   **SUPERFICIAL PULSE**

Heart ·············· ············ Small Intestine

Liver ······················· ······· Gall Bladder

Kidney ·················· ········ Bladder

LEFT

DEEP PULSE   **SUPERFICIAL PULSE**

Lungs ············ ········· Colon

Spleen ··············· ············· Stomach

Circulation ················ ······ Triple Heater

RIGHT

THE TWELVE PULSES

TAKING PULSES

Although pulse diagnosis was used prior to A.D. 400, it was not widespread in ancient China until that time. Having evolved over time, pulse diagnosis can be compared to Western diagnostic tests—X rays, laboratory tests, EKGs. In a healthy person the pulses move smoothly; when there is an imbalance in the body, pulses can become choppy, slippery, wiry, blocked, to name a few characteristics. There are twelve pulses, each one relating to a different organ system. A skilled practitioner can tell a great deal about a patient by the quality of his or her pulse.

THE CHINESE TEN ASKING SONGS

Developed over centuries of practice, the ten asking songs are actually categories of inquiry that Traditional Chinese Medicine (TCM) practitioners and acupuncturists use as a very important diagnostic tool.

1. *Chills or fever* The severity and frequency of fever and chills are keys to determining yin and yang deficiencies and whether an illness is on the interior or exterior of the body. For example, if a patient has an illness that has been present for an extended period of time and is characterized by an intolerance of cold, a preference for warmth, and no fever, there may be a yang deficiency.

2. *Perspiration* The presence or absence of perspiration, when perspiration occurs, and how much and where on the body it occurs, are all important clues for the practitioner making a diagnosis.

3. *Pain* Chinese practitioners focus on many aspects of pain including the time of its onset, how long it lasts, and the type of pain, outlined as follows:

   - *Dull pain* can be attributed to an irregular flow of qi and blood.
   - *Stabbing pain* can be the result of a stagnation of blood.
   - *Burning pain* can point to an excess of yang heat and a yin deficiency.
   - *Gaseous pain* indicates an obstruction of the flow of qi.
   - *Distending pain* can be a result of stagnant qi.

   After determining the type of pain, the practitioner probes further to discover more about the pain: Is it accompanied by other symptoms? Is it in the head, limbs, or trunk? How long are the episodes, and when do they occur?

4. *Sensations in the abdomen and chest* Is there any pain or discomfort?

5. *Bowel and urine habits, consistency and color of products of elimination*

6. *Appetite* Has it increased or decreased? Do you have cravings? What do you crave?

7. *Thirst* Are you thirsty? Has your thirst increased or decreased? Has the time of day when you get thirsty changed?

8. *Hearing* Do you experience any ringing or unusual sounds in your ears? Any hearing loss? Any breaks in hearing?

9. *Previous history of disease* Is there a history of disease or ailments in your family? Does the family history worry you?

10. *The onset and development of the present illness* The practitioner asks detailed questions to get to the root of the illness.

READING THE TONGUE

In both Eastern and Western diagnosis, a light red tongue with a thin white covering generally indicates a normal healthy person. Inspected for general color, shape, and type of coating, the tongue can provide practitioners with clear clues to the roots of illness. The general color of the tongue is very important to the Eastern practitioner, revealing the strength of qi and the body's vitality. Other important clues are found on the tongue by examining the shape and surface: flabby, swollen, thin, cracked, containing teeth imprints, covered with phlegm, and flaccid, to name a few.

Eastern Treatments

ACUPUNCTURE

Used to restore balance to the body, acupuncture needling began gaining acceptance in this country, as mentioned earlier, after *New York Times* reporter, James Reston, was given acupuncture needling for postsurgical pain following an emergency appendectomy while

WHAT THE TONGUE CAN TELL US

TONGUE	WESTERN ANALYSIS	EASTERN ANALYSIS
A PALE TONGUE	A pale tongue could indicate a decrease in the blood volume or circulation. Such conditions as anemia, hypoproteinemia, disorders of the digestive system, low basal rate of metabolism, or inadequate glandular secretions could be evidenced by a pale tongue.	A yang qi deficiency and insufficiency of blood and qi are often indicated by a pale tongue. An Eastern practitioner, much like a Western doctor, would take other diagnostic measures before making a definitive diagnosis.
A DEEP RED TONGUE	A deep red tongue could reflect such things as dehydration, febrile diseases, any one of a number of serious liver conditions, advanced cancer, or coma.	A deep red tongue is a sign of severe internal heat, seen in those suffering from fevers.
A PURPLE TONGUE	Circulatory disturbances, lowered blood oxygen, cancer, liver disease, heart problems, or alcoholism— all can be represented by a purple tongue.	A purple tongue indicates stagnation of blood and sometimes an irregular flow of qi. Circulatory disturbances, lowered blood oxygen, cancer, liver disease, heart problems, or alcoholism may also be among the conditions considered in an Eastern analysis of a purple tongue.

covering a story in China in the 1970s. Since that time acupuncture has been gaining acceptance in the Western world, and for more than a decade the World Health Organization has recognized that such things as bronchitis, flu, arthritis, stroke, infertility, dizziness, insomnia, and depression respond to acupuncture needling therapy. Studies during this time have also shown acupuncture to be highly effective for treating people with alcohol and drug dependency in conjunction with treatment programs. Recovering addicts treated with acupuncture had a much lower recidivism rate than those who were not.[2] Acupuncture has also been effective in treating other addictions such as cigarette smoking and overeating.

Misinformed people often think that acupuncture needling is the only component of acupuncture therapy, when in fact the acupuncturist employs many Oriental and herbal treatments and philosophies in helping patients. In this country, acupuncturists are still restricted by current laws, and in many states they are not able to treat patients without a medical doctor's prescription. Nevertheless, in November 1997, the National Institutes of Health recognized acupuncture treatments for a variety of conditions.

Following a lengthy diagnostic procedure, taking into account the patient's life and sorrows and involving the reading of the pulses and the inspection of the tongue, the acupuncturist makes a diagnosis and develops a prescription of treatment, which often includes needling. When needling is part of the prescription, the accupuncturist selects a set of impulse points along the body's meridians, which correspond with the organs needing attention. The treatment makes use of selected gates and doors. The needle acts as the opener or closer, summoning, allowing, pushing, pulling the energy to and from one pathway to another.

ACUPUNCTURE LICENSING

To become a licensed acupuncturist in the United States, a practitioner is required to complete more than 2,400 hours of clinical training and practice. A Western medical doctor, in comparison, is required to take only 200 hours of training for certification. This difference in standards worries many acupuncturists, as acupuncture treatment requires an extremely skilled practitioner, and many believe that 200 hours of training is not adequate for treating patients.

Acupuncture Points There are over 350 acupuncture points on the body, and charts designed thousands of years ago are still available to guide practitioners along the meridians or body channels. But for centuries, traditional Chinese practitioners have been able to find exact points by probing with their fingers, recognizing individual points by touch. Patients experienced in acupuncture are also often able to feel the point. According to several acupuncturists, the acupuncture or impulse points often feel like elastic-bordered depressions in the skin. Most of the points on the back and extremities can be located by touch, but there are those on the front of the body, like those on the abdomen and face, that cannot be found by this method. Measurement is required. But measurement is not done using some sort of tool; rather the practitioner finds a reference point on the patient's body near the approximate location of the acupuncture point and finds the exact location by taking a measurement using the patient's bodily proportions. Jody Forman, a licensed acupuncturist at the former Dogwood Institute in Charlottesville, Virginia, says that to find the more hard-to-define points it is important for the practitioner to measure distances using the patient's fingers or body parts, not the practitioner's. Interestingly, each practitioner discovers the path to healing in slightly different ways. And each healer's descriptions of the process vary, just as patient tales of the needling and qi movement unfold in terms of their own individual experiences. But no matter what the description or the variations in the process, the heart of acupuncture therapy is restoring balance to the body.

Acupuncture Needles There are many sizes and types of acupuncture needles. Acupuncturist Jody Forman says that she almost always uses Japanese needles because they are very thin and hairlike. Jody, who studied in China, says that the Chinese use much larger needles, and they often laugh at the fine needles used in America. "They asked me how do we get any effect with such small needles, but I know if we used those big needles in this country, nobody would ever get acupuncture," she says, laughing and admitting that acupuncture in this country has been Americanized. The Japanese acupuncture needle is coated, and according to Jody, this makes the insertion quick and relatively painless. She uses an insertion device, a small plastic tube, which she says keeps her insertions consistent. The needles used by most acupuncturists today are disposable, so there is no risk of infection with HIV or other contaminants.

The typical patient has anywhere from four to twenty needles inserted in a treatment session. According to Jody, one session does not effect a cure; often a patient needs to be treated several times to realize results.

> *"Acupuncture takes time. It works on a subtle level, working with the qi, coaxing it to move. In China the people who work for the government go to the doctor everyday for about ten days. In America, people often come to an acupuncturist with chronic conditions, after they have exhausted Western methods. It has been a longstanding problem, and it takes time for discernible changes. I tell my clients that it will take at least ten visits."*

> —Jody Forman, M.S.W., M.O.A.M., a licensed
> acupuncturist, who has studied in China

What to Expect When You Visit an Acupuncturist Most first visits with acupuncturists, which usually involve much more than needling, last about two hours and cost somewhere between $75 and $125, depending on the location, type of practitioner, and state laws governing acupuncture practice. During the first visit the relationship is established as the acupuncturist or other Eastern practitioner delves into the patient's physical, emotional, and spiritual beliefs and life difficulties. Depending on the nature of the problem being treated, one usually visits the acupuncturist six to twelve times. As one acupuncturist told me, this discovery process is much like an elegant song that guides the dance between the practitioner and the patient.

COTTON SHIRTS, SILK SHIRTS

Jody Forman says that the Chinese often refer to Americans as "silk shirts," because the Chinese believe that people in this country require a much gentler acupuncture approach because we are more fragile. The Chinese view themselves as cotton shirts, because they are hearty stock: working outdoors, their skin is tougher, and because of their stronger constitution, they are able to withstand a more aggressive acupuncture approach.

First-of-Its-Kind Survey of Acupuncture Users In 1996 Claire Cassidy, Ph.D., medical anthropologist, conducted a survey of 575 acupuncture users from six clinics in five states under the umbrella of the Traditional Acupuncture Institute in Columbia, Maryland. Acupuncture in this case refers to an Eastern blended model of treatment that goes beyond acupuncture needling.[3] Here are the results:

- 91.5 percent of those surveyed reported the disappearance or improvement of symptoms following acupuncture treatment.
- 84 percent said they see their conventional MDs less often because of acupuncture.
- 79 percent said that they use fewer prescription drugs as a result of their acupuncture.
- 77.7 percent said that some of their symptoms or complaints had improved.
- 77.5 percent said that they were seeing a physical therapist less because of their acupuncture treatments.
- 77 percent reported that they were asking for fewer reimbursements from their insurance company.
- 70 percent of those to whom surgery had been recommended said they had avoided it through acupuncture.
- 63 percent reported that they used acupuncture to keep them healthy.
- 58.5 percent said they were seeing a psychotherapist less because of acupuncture treatments.
- 7.8 percent named symptoms or conditions that had not changed with acupuncture.
- 0.7 percent said that their symptoms or complaints had gotten worse.

Table 1: Clinics Participating in the Survey

Clinic Name/ Clinic Location	Type of Clinic	Acupuncture Style
Centre for Traditional Acupuncture Columbia, Md.	Private	Five-Element
Ruscombe Mansion Baltimore, Md.	Private	Five-Element
New England School of Acupuncture Boston, Mass.	School	TCM/Japanese
Northwest Institute of Acupuncture Seattle, Wash.	School	TCM
Oriental Medicine Gipson Speciality Center Memphis, Tenn.	Private	TCM
Chinese Medicine Works San Francisco	Private	Eclectic

*Five-Element: a form of Chinese Medicine.
TCM: Traditional Chinese Medicine.
Eclectic: Varying styles of acupuncture.

Table 2: How Respondents Describe Their Experience

"For each sentence check the word that best describes your experience with acupuncture."

| | PERCENTAGES | | | |
	NONE	A LITTLE	SOME	MOST
I feel better	0.4	2.3	21.1	76.2
I can work better	1.6	4.5	30.2	63.6
I have more energy	1.1	6.4	34.3	58.2
I am more focused	1.2	7.4	33.3	58.2
I have less pain	1.9	5.9	28.4	63.8
I miss fewer work days	9.4	3.0	16.6	71.0
I get along better with others	2.3	4.8	24.1	68.8

Survey data received from Claire Cassidy, Ph.D., medical anthropologist, 1996. Traditional Acupuncture Institute, Columbia, Md.

Table 3: Comparing Costs for Biomedical Treatment Versus Acupuncture Treatment

	BIOMEDICAL COSTS	ACUPUNCTURE COSTS
Average Number of Visits (in three months)	6.0	2.2
Average Total Cost	$409.09	$264.40

Survey data received from Claire Cassidy, Ph.D., medical anthropologist, 1996. Traditional Acupuncture Institute, Columbia, Md.

> *"I can get my cortisone covered, prescription pain meds covered. I can get a $1,500 MRI and get reimbursed, and what does an MRI do to make me better? But the only thing that works for me are my acupuncture treatments, which are less than $50 and I can't get that covered. I think it's my constitutional right to decide about the path of my healing journey."*
>
> —Arlene Stillwater, 54

> *"I was referred to an acupuncturist by my homeopathic doctor for chronic shoulder pain. Since I was going through a depression around the same time, my acupuncturist offered treatment for my moods as well (which I didn't know was possible). I gratefully accepted and continued those treatments, which helped me eventually to take charge of my life again. Both symptoms have long since disappeared."*
>
> —Female, 41-50 age group, survey respondent

Cupping Cupping is an ancient Chinese therapy designed to help move qi and promote the free flow of blood and qi along the body's energy channels. Often used to dispel cold and dampness, cupping is indicated for the treatment of conditions caused predominantly by wind dampness: lower back pain, joint pain in the shoulders and legs, gastrointestinal difficulties such as vomiting and diarrhea, and lung problems associated with cough and asthma.

Before the process begins, the patient lies facedown, barebacked, on a table. Often massage tables are used. Dome-shaped glass, bamboo, or pottery jars are prepared for this technique. The practitioner holds a cotton ball in a hemostat (a tweezer-like tool), soaks it in alcohol, and, while holding the cup close to the back, lights the cotton ball, passing the flame quickly into the jar, releasing the oxygen. The jar is quickly turned down onto the patient's back, creating a vacuum. The jar sticks to the skin, sucking a bubble of skin into its center. The more stagnant the patient's qi, the more purple the bubble appears. Depending on the practitioner, the jars are either left in place for ten to fifteen minutes or moved on the back, with the practitioner taking care not to cross over the spine. Patients describe the sensation of cupping as strange or unusual, but few complain of pain.

There are some precautions that should be followed in cupping. It is not advisable to use cups for patients with high fevers; or to apply the cups to the abdominal or sacral (literally the last bone of the spine) regions of pregnant women; or to use cupping if the patient is susceptible to spontaneous bleeding or has difficulty stopping bleeding after trauma. Some patients will experience a blood stasis or bruise to the area that has been cupped. The discoloration generally disappears after several days, and occasionally the heated jar will cause blisters to form on the skin.

Moxibustion Another healing art, moxibustion involves the application of a heated herb to acupuncture points along the body's meridians. This treatment can involve several different methods of burning dried mugwort leaves, known as *moxa,* and placing them directly or indirectly on the skin. If the herb is to be applied directly, dried moxa wool rolled into a cone is placed on the skin and lit. Once the patient feels the heat, the moxa cone is extinguished. Indirect applications can take several forms: prerolled moxa sticks are lit and held close to the skin; moxa can be placed on slices of ginger or garlic and burned. Ginger helps circulation.

Moxa is used to treat many symptoms and ailments, such as fatigue, cold, back problems, stiff neck, or a frozen shoulder.

Chinese Remedial Massage Known as *tuina* or *an-mo,* these techniques either tonify or soothe the system. Through rubbing or pressing hand motions (an-mo) or thrusting and rolling hand motions (tuina), both systems of treatment use a complex series of hand movements to produce the desired healing effects.

THREE

East/West Approaches to Treatment: Chronic Maladies

"I was referred to an acupuncturist by my doctor for my asthma. I was on a breathing machine and prednisone; I had suffered with this condition for more than 20 years. I spent $1,000's of dollars every year on hospitals and ambulances and medicine. After four treatments, I am off the breathing machine, off almost all of my medicines. I feel 26 right now."

—Mary Jane Heffner, 64

ALLERGIES, HAY FEVER, AND SINUS PROBLEMS

A Western Approach

As we enter allergy season, many people feel the discomfort of pollen-filled air. And for the nearly 35 million seasonal allergy sufferers, itchy and watery eyes, sneezing, and a runny nose are a way of life in the spring and fall. But for individuals with chronic allergies and sinus problems, headaches and postnasal drip can be a daily annoyance, and many times something other than pollen is the culprit. It's not uncommon for those suffering from allergy symptoms to blame the headaches and nasal congestion on allergies, often self-medicating with over-the-counter remedies. Western doctors say that these symptoms, left untreated, can lead to sinus infections, which require antibiotic treatment. Individuals with chronic allergy symptoms may discover that they are actually allergic to dust, mold, or even the family pet. And although we cannot prevent allergies, we can avoid some (I can't possibly avoid my pet) known allergens once they have been identified. When an allergen is not avoidable and the reaction becomes serious or incapacitating, many Western doctors advise that the patient receive immunotherapy—allergy shots—to desensitize the body to the known substance.

An Eastern Approach

Hay fever is usually viewed as a wind heat invasion of the lungs. Eastern doctors treat this malady very simply and generally effectively. By opening the lung qi, through acupuncture needling, the wind heat is expelled from the body. Herbs can also be used, including chrysanthemum flowers, mulberry leaves, ephedra, and cinnamon twigs. Sinus problems, on the other hand, are seen as connected to a lung qi deficiency and damp heat. In addition to acupuncture needling, peppermint, tangerine peel, xanthium fruit, and fritillary bulbs are often used.

Ayurvedic Herbal Tea for Sinus Problems

I have been plagued by sinus problems since I was a child, and drinking this tea three times a day keeps me relatively free from sinus headache. The tea consists of all of these herbs: ginger root, licorice root, peppermint leaf, anise seed, tulsi leaf, gotu kola, skullcap root, cardamon seed, eucalyptus leaf, orange peel, black pepper, clove bud, cinnamon bark, amla extract, angelica root, magnolia flower, peony root, and poria cocos fungus. In many healthfood stores it's known as Allergy Season Tea.

Other Options for Treating Allergies, Hay Fever, and Sinus Problems

- Apply pressure in the webbed area between the thumb and index finger for several minutes (a point called the enclosed valley).
- Massage lavender oil into the temples.
- Increase vitamin C intake through supplements or eating more citrus fruits.
- Take vitamin B supplements.
- Reduce your intake of dairy.
- Do steam inhalation using eucalyptus or pine essential oils or apply mentholatum under the nose.
- Explore homeopathic remedies: silica, pulsatilla, and kali bich.

Consult an acupuncturist, herbalist, or homeopathic practitioner for information on doses and treatments.

CARPAL TUNNEL SYNDROME

A Western Approach

Carpal tunnel syndrome, which often affects middle-aged women or individuals with an underactive thyroid or diabetes, is a result of a pinched nerve in the wrist area. Numbness and tingling in the thumb, index and middle fingers are symptoms often associated with carpal tunnel syndrome. Some patients may experience wrist pain radiating all the way up the arm to the shoulder. Frequently these symptoms become worse at night and when driving. There is much confusion about the cause of the ailment; media accounts often blame carpal tunnel syndrome on the use of computer keyboards. But many Western doctors dispute this information, saying there is no evidence to support this theory. In the Western world, the cause of carpal tunnel syndrome remains disputed.

According to Western views, this often painful condition results from pressure on the median nerve at the point where it passes into the hand through the carpal tunnel, which is actually a gap under a ligament at the front of the wrist. Because carpal tunnel syndrome can be confused with other conditions, diagnosis is determined only after the doctor takes a medical history and does a physical exam. Often-times Western doctors use an electrical nerve conduction study, referred to as an EMG, to test the median nerve. Treatment is prescribed based on the severity of the condition. Frequently the symptoms of the pressure on the nerve can be alleviated through the use of wrist splints. If symptoms persist, doctors may prescribe corti-sone injections to the area. Only after more conservative measures fail is surgery suggested. An operation cuts the carpal tunnel ligament, relieving pressure on the nerve.

An Eastern Approach

Carpal tunnel syndrome is viewed by Eastern practitioners as signify-ing the presence of cold and damp in the affected region. Acupuncture needling, along with moxibustion and herbal treatment, is often used to alleviate the problem. Some practitioners may also use cupping. Dried moxa wool can also be rolled into a cone and placed directly on the skin and lit. Once heat is felt, the moxa cone is extinguished. Indirect applications can take several forms: pre-rolled moxa sticks are lit and held close to the skin; can be placed on slices of ginger or garlic and burned. Ginger helps circulation. Herbal remedies are sometimes prescribed to be taken as a tea. The ingredients are cinnamon twigs, mulberry twigs, angelica root, and white ginger.

Other Options for Treating Carpal Tunnel Syndrome

- Alternately apply hot and cold compresses to the affected area.
- Take high doses of vitamin B6 and magnesium (consult your practitioner for advice on the number of milligrams).
- Seek out osteopathic manipulation.
- Try massage treatments.
- Ask your practitioner about homeopathic remedies, including Traumeel.

Consult an acupuncturist, herbalist, or homeopathic practitioner for more information on these treatments.

CHRONIC FATIGUE SYNDROME

A Western Approach

There is much debate in Western medicine about chronic fatigue; some practitioners believe the collection of symptoms and ailments that fall under this syndrome have a mental or emotional root and that there is no real illness. Doctors who have this mind-set put forward the following arguments: there are no observable markers for identifying the presence of the ailment; no cause has been found; and lack of access to recent clinical findings.

More than 70 percent of those suffering from chronic fatigue syndrome are women. Some of the symptoms are mental fogginess, excessive fatigue, general pain, headache, sore throat, and sleep problems. Stress appears to trigger these symptoms. Some preliminary Western research indicates that the disorder may be viral in origin; other studies point to genetics and environmental factors. Possible treatments vary at this time, but it is not uncommon for Western doctors to treat the symptoms with antidepressants such as Prozac and amitriptyline (a tricyclic antidepressant) and anti-inflammatories to alleviate the pain. At this time, conventional Western medicine offers little comfort to those with chronic fatigue syndrome.

An Eastern Approach

In Eastern cultures, chronic fatigue syndrome is often referred to as tired all the time syndrome, and the causes are seen as varying from depression to underlying physical illness. The Eastern practitioner will determine whether the cause is emotional or physical by examining the pulse and tongue and other physical indicators in addition to taking a lengthy history and considering environmental factors as well. Once premenstrual syndrome, menopause, or other hormonal imbalances are ruled out for women, as well as thyroid problems or Addison's disease, the practitioner treats the chronic fatigue as a qi deficiency. If the patient is tired and feeling cold, the problem is a yang deficiency. If tired and hot, it is a yin deficiency. Herbal remedies, such as ginseng, goldenseal and echinacea, along with acupuncture needling, massage, and qigong (a therapeutic set of exercises) are generally prescribed.

Other Options for Treating Chronic Fatigue Syndrome

- Try meditation and yoga.
- Avoid processed foods, sugars, alcohol, and caffeine. Concentrate on consuming a lot of slow-release carbohydrates, such as pasta and lots of bananas.
- Engage in exercise like walking or stretching.
- Get at least six to eight hours of sleep per night.
- Take baths with lavender, grapefruit, rosemary, juniper, marjoram herbs, or essential oils.
- Take oil of evening primrose supplements.
- Take vitamin B-complex, zinc, and vitamin C.
- Seek out support groups.

Consult an acupuncturist, herbalist, or homeopathic practitioner for more detailed doses.

MÉNIÈRE'S DISEASE

A Western Approach

Ménière's disease, which, according to the Western view, is caused by an increase in the pressure of fluids in the inner ear, can be debilitating for those suffering from its effects.

Fluids in the chambers of the inner ear are constantly produced and absorbed by the circulatory system, and any disturbance to this delicate balance can cause increased fluid pressure and dizziness. In most people, ear infections or allergies can upset this balance temporarily, but for those with Ménière's disease increased pressure in the inner ear is a permanent problem. If left untreated, the symptoms can become violent. The onset of an attack is characterized by repeated episodes of dizziness, hearing loss, and a roaring, buzzing, or ringing sound in the ear; these attacks can last from one to several hours and are often accompanied by nausea and vomiting.

Western doctors believe it is important to determine whether attacks of vertigo are Ménière's disease, and once they diagnose the disorder, treatment can begin. Although there is currently no cure for Ménière's disease in Western medicine, the attacks of vertigo that are a common and frequent part of the disease can be controlled in nearly all cases. For some patients a fluid pill and a low- sodium diet will reduce the amount of fluid that accumulates in the ear, relieving the pressure and dizziness. For others vitamins, antihistamines, and steroids offer relief. In some cases the vertigo cannot be controlled by conservative treatment, so surgery is required. Several surgical techniques are available, including a decompression procedure, in which an endolymphatic shunt is implanted; vestibular neurectomy, in which the balance nerve is cut; and labyrinthectomy, a procedure in which the balance and hearing functions are destroyed in one ear.

An Eastern Approach

In Traditional Chinese Medicine, Ménière's disease is often seen as signifying kidney weakness, because the kidneys are linked with the ear. With kidney deficiency there is internal cold, and the fluid processed by the kidneys, under normal conditions, becomes mucus or phlegm. Because of the kidney weakness, the spleen also becomes weak. According to Chinese teachings, the excess fluid goes to the ears, the brain fails to get proper nourishment, which in turn leads to dizziness and loss of balance. To help the patient, Chinese practitioners would recommend treatment that warms and tonifies the kidneys and strengthens the spleen. Some of the herbs that might be prescribed include a combination of astragalus, ginseng, orange peel, ginger or cinnamon bark, and dong quai. Or a brothy soup of herbs used as a tonic might be prescribed.

People with Ménière's disease are advised to avoid cold foods such as salads, cold drinks, ice cream, sugar, and dairy products, which tend to increase dampness in the body and produce more fluids. Acupuncture needling could also be part of the treatment.

Consult an acupuncturist, herbalist, or homeopathic practitioner for more information on possible treatments.

MENOPAUSE

A Western Approach

Menopause is part of the natural progression of a woman's life, and generally it begins its gradual course when a woman reaches her late forties or early fifties, although the age and onset vary. Menopause is a time when a woman passes from the reproductive to nonreproductive years of life. In the years or months leading up to menopause, the ovaries' production of estrogen slows, often causing hormones to fluctuate. Menstrual periods become irregular, and some women may also experience insomnia, hot flashes, night sweats, depression, frequent urination or urinary incontinence, vaginal dryness, and a change in sexual desire. Although the majority of women experience some or all of the signs and symptoms of menopause, some women have no symptoms at all. As hormone levels decrease, Western doctors believe that bone loss occurs, so it is important to receive some type of hormone replacement therapy to counter bone loss.

An Eastern Approach

In Eastern cultures menopause is viewed as a natural progression in a woman's life. Seasonal cycles and the incidence of menopausal problems in Asian women is greatly diminished compared to American women. If problems such as hot flashes, mood swings, or vaginal dryness do arise, they are often considered to be signs of an imbalance in the body. Acupuncture needling is often very effective in treating these problems. And occasionally herbal treatment is also used to restore hormonal balance. Some herbs that are used are angelica root, peony root, and raw and cooked rehmannia.

Other Options for Treating Menopausal Ailments

- Take supplements, including oil of evening primrose, magnesium, zinc, iron, and vitamin B-complex and vitamins C and E.
- Indulge yourself with lemongrass baths.
- Follow a diet regime low in caffeine and high in soy products, such as tofu, tempei, and soy milk.
- Use jojoba oil to alleviate vaginal dryness prior to intercourse.
- Put a few drops of rose essential oil or diluted tea tree oil in your bath water.
- Try meditation, exercise, and yoga.

Consult an acupuncturist, herbalist, or homeopathic practitioner for more details on doses and treatments.

TEMPOROMANDIBULAR JOINT DISORDER (TMJ/TMD)

A Western Approach

Temporomandibular joint syndrome (TMJ), now commonly referred to as temporomandibular disorder (TMD), occurs 80 percent of the time in females between the ages of twenty-five and forty-five. This often painful condition can affect the jaw joint or the muscles, tendons, and ligaments surrounding the joint. The disorder is characterized most frequently by an inability to open the mouth, pain in the jaw joints, and pain or spasms of the facial head muscles used for chewing. Commonly the condition is caused by clenching or grinding the teeth; an improperly aligned bite; or an injury to the neck, head, or jaw. This category of TMD can often be treated with conservative, nonsurgical methods. Treatment involves the application of heat to the affected area, the use of anti-inflammatory medications, muscle relaxants, and a soft diet. The patient may also be fitted with a plastic splint to cushion the bite, which relaxes the muscles and protects the teeth. Physical therapy and biofeedback have also proved very helpful in treating this type of TMD.

A small percentage of individuals with TMD have degenerative joint disease, and they may require surgical intervention. The surgical technique varies depending on the severity of the disease, but many times simple outpatient procedures can correct the disorder. In more severe arthritic conditions, however, the joint may require more advanced surgical techniques. Sometimes a total joint replacement is required.

An Eastern Approach

Although they do not call the disorder TMJ/TMD, Eastern practitioners treat patients complaining of teeth grinding. They also believe this behavior leads to disorders of the joints and jaws. Sometimes the condition is thought to be caused by too much heat in the spleen and stomach, which often becomes worse at night. Treatments include methods for cooling the heat. Herbal medicines used for this purpose include Chinese yam, golden thread, lotus seeds, or skullcap.

Other Options for Treating TMJ/TMD

- Try practicing meditation and yoga to promote relaxation and internal healing.
- Apply ice packs on the affected jaw area.
- Try exercises designed to relieve muscle tension in the jaw, which can include autogenic training or biofeedback.
- Consult a homeopathic practitioner about the following medicines: Arsenicum alb., phytolacca, zinc, cina, or santoninum.

Consult an acupuncturist, herbalist, or homeopathic practitioner for more details on doses and treatments.

FOUR

East/West Approaches to Treatment: 20th-Century Killers

"I remember this patient who came to the clinic up until the week he died. He didn't seem sick. He just kept coming in for his treatments. This was a last chance for him. He had resigned himself to the fact that he was going to die. He wasn't talking cure. He was talking a better way of life."

—Howard Moffett, former director of the
American College of Traditional Chinese Medicine, San Francisco

HIV/AIDS

It was a cold, damp fall day. About ten of us—some dressed in faded jeans, others in heels, dramatically veiled hats and black chiffon—carried out buckets of water and shovels to the carefully selected site on an old Virginia farm. Overlooking rows of blue-tinged mountains and a pastoral countryside dotted with black and white cows grazing as if tomorrow would never come, the eclectic caravan moved deliberately, the rising and falling of our measured breaths muffled under the crunching leaves. The solemn procession advanced without words—a rare occurrence for this group of friends. Once inside the aging, gated space, we all stopped, avoiding each other's gaze, hoping our internal sorrow was not evident. And as the first shovel was thrust into the red clay, the sound of metal scraping stone pierced our hearts. A circle formed and one by one we dug a piece of the earth, the hole growing ever deeper, until the flowering pear was carried to its place of honor. Gently placing nature's gift in its new home between the giant maple and the fading, marred cornerstones, we nourished the sapling with the water we had lovingly carried from the barn. After what seemed like an eternity of stillness, one friend placed the red clay back over the fresh opening, covering the roots. A blanket of comfort, protection. Holding hands we chanted, our songs reaching the heavens. Slowly, one by one we paid tribute to our friend whose life would continue through the flowering pear. David was full of life. Handsome, young, and irreverently funny. Now gone. He died alone, of AIDS. Perhaps a little late, we gathered to pay tribute to a life lived fully.

David never told us he had AIDS. But we all knew. We silently watched his ankles turn purple and swell. We looked the other way as his clothes began to bag, and his cheekbones defined his sallow skin. Trying to protect his privacy and our own fears, we never said anything. Our silence kept him from us. We helped him build a wall, pushing him into exile and perhaps making his own fears of dying alone a reality. Perhaps it was denial. Or maybe David really wanted it that way, to go quickly. We will never know.

Worldwide there are more than 28 million people infected with the HIV virus, according to the most recent World Health Organization's data. Despite our technologically advanced culture, a cure eludes medical researchers, and the cost of care continues to soar. Nonetheless, there are those who have defied the odds. There are those who say AIDS is not the death sentence it's made out to be. One such person is San Francisco-based AIDS activist George Wedemeyer, a fifty-five-year-old U.S. Department of Labor investigator who has been fighting for his life since 1985. And so far he's winning.

> *"AIDS is not the death sentence if you know how to take of yourself. And I credit Traditional Chinese Medicine and Qigong with my survival."*
>
> —George Wedemeyer, San Francisco, diagnosed HIV-positive in 1985

> *"The new understanding of the AIDS virus is that it is never dormant. It is always a tug of war. That is how the Chinese viewed it all along. The virus will always be there and will always replicate. It is only when the body is weakened that it gets the upper hand."*
>
> —Howard Moffett spearheaded one of the first California studies on AIDS and Chinese Medicine

AIDS Activist Outliving Predictions

When doctors told George Wedemeyer he had AIDS, he initially rejected AZT and most of the other advice he was given. Although now he blends Western and Eastern treatments in keeping his disease at bay. He saw his friends taking the potent anti-viral and getting worse and dying. George admits that his doctor warned he was flirting with disaster, but George says that he had researched his options carefully and knew what he was doing. "I investigated Chinese medicine and compared it to Western medicine. I made my choice wisely." He works out at the gym, something doctors told him to stop doing. He takes a dozen or so Chinese herbs and has regular acupuncture sessions, treatments doctors told him were of unproven use. He practices the gentle Chinese art of qigong, which he says keeps him alive. Studying qigong (pronounced chee-gung) as part of his treatment regimen, George says that within two months he could feel the difference.

Moving from San Diego to San Francisco, he met up with T'ai-Chi (pronounced tye jee) instructor Emelio Gonzalez, who is also HIV-positive. And after a short time, the two developed a gentler approach to the qigong movements, one that is not too rigorous for those who are sick. And in 1990 they began to co-teach these healing, graceful movements to others. In the beginning, they offered the classes for free and now ask a $1 donation per class for those with HIV, cancer, and other chronic or life-threatening diseases, and $5 for anyone else.

According to Traditional Chinese Medicine, health is restored when the body's qi is flowing and balanced. Qigong gentle exercises are actually slow, fluid movements which reduce stress and are designed to balance the body's energy along the meridians, which correspond to the body's organs and emotions. George and Emelio have incorporated such things as the Six Healing Sounds (the use of sound, color, and movement) and Tiger Mountain (T'ai-Chi postures in a qigong stance) to help balance and heal organ systems in the body.

Now, twelve years later, George is still following his Chinese Medicine routine, never misses a morning of his own twenty-minute healing qigong ritual, he sees an acupuncturist twice a week, and he's added a mainstream doctor to his list of practitioners. And even though his white blood cell count has remained dangerously low over the past decade, George is living life to the fullest. He continues to work at a frantic pace. He's helped push legislation in favor of alternative therapies, he's gaining a national reputation for his work with other AIDS patients, he speaks at international AIDS conferences, and, along with Emelio, he still teaches qigong classes to people with AIDS and cancer in San Francisco.

The San Francisco Community Health Clinic

The nation's first federally funded alternative medicine HIV public health clinic project got underway in 1992 after the San Francisco County Department of Public Health joined forces with the California-based American College of Traditional Chinese Medicine. In the first-of-its-kind U.S.-based project, people with symptomatic HIV infection were offered access to acupuncture and Chinese herbs in an attempt to allay the discomfort of traditional Western therapies such as the antiviral AZT, and to improve the patient's quality of life. Falling under the Ryan White Comprehensive AIDS Resources Emergency (CARE) Act of Congress, the project was funded with both local government and federal dollars and was administered under the direction of the San Francisco Department of Public Health AIDS Office. According to Howard Moffett, then director of the American College of Traditional Chinese Medicine, this venture was a major treatment turning point for people with HIV, since this type of government assistance had never before been available for alternative therapies. Moffett, a licensed acupuncturist and researcher who is now studying public health systems at Harvard, says that he hopes the San Francisco Clinic and its findings will pave the way for alternative public health clinics throughout the nation. Nonetheless, he acknowledges that the controversy that continues over the efficacy of Eastern treatments, and in particular traditional Chinese medicine, does not bode well for future funding.

The San Francisco project now treads a fine line, continually threatened with losing funds. And although not part of the clinic's original design, patients must now use Western physicians as gate-keepers for referral for acupuncture and herbs. But while the funding remains in place, people with HIV can receive free acupuncture treatments, something that Moffett says is only part of the prescription. It's helping people live with grace, even if there is no cure.

Recalling the story of one patient, Moffett says, "I remember this patient who came to the clinic up until the week he died. He didn't seem sick. He just kept coming in for his treatments. This was a last chance for him. He had resigned himself to the fact that he was going to die. He wasn't talking cure. He was talking a better way of life." And Chinese medicine, which helps people function at a higher level, does just that. According to Moffett, practicing Chinese medicine is like tending your garden. It takes work and patience to cultivate good health, and Chinese medicine focuses on the person, not the disease.

At the San Francisco-based public health clinics, as at most acupuncture clinics in this country, the patient gets individualized attention; Moffett and others agree that this level of care is crucial to healing. Patients aren't treated with what has come to be a Western medicine managed care buzzword, best practices—across-the-board standards of treating certain conditions; they are treated with concern for who they are as individuals, and care plans are based on patients' lifestyle and needs.

Some of the patients seeking treatment at the HIV health clinics use only Chinese medicine, but many combine therapies. According to Moffett, it is important to understand the complexity of the patient and his or her individual situation, including learning about his or her living environment. According to Moffett, there are many patients who are seeking alternatives to the antivirals like AZT. You have to take the time to talk to them, to build a level of trust, let them feel more comfortable before they will disclose what they are going through, he says. He admits that Chinese medicine is a lot like nursing—dealing with human responses with care and compassion, and relating to the patient. But, says Moffett and others, giving that amount of time to someone—something that managed care won't allow in traditional Western medical practices—is the key. It's touching the patient, getting to his or her feelings and needs, that helps bring about positive changes in the patient's life.

Since the inception of the HIV Clinic program, response has been overwhelming, and there are never less than a hundred people on the waiting list for services. First contacting individuals in their target population—the Asian, Latino, and African-American communities—practitioners and researchers broke this population into three groups: (1) people who could not tolerate standard drug therapy and needed access to safe, nontoxic alternatives; (2) people for whom immune suppressing therapies were counterproductive; and (3) people who needed relief from the side effects of other medical treatments.[1]

Patients were then seen by practitioners predominantly trained in China. Although the patients had already been diagnosed in the Western medical system, the patients received an in-depth Eastern diagnosis, which gave the practitioners a prescription guide. According to initial research findings, which were led by Moffett, the most common Eastern-based diagnoses seen in the AIDS population that visited the clinic were spleen qi deficiency, which is a digestive functioning impairment and may manifest in loss of appetite, diarrhea, abdominal distention, nausea, vomiting, and weight loss (the spleen helps with digestion and assimilation of food nutrients); liver qi congestion, which means that physical or emotional tensions may impede the smooth flow of qi, and the accompanying symptoms may include irritability, headaches, visual disturbances, flank pain (the liver spreads qi); and general qi and yin deficiency.[2] Patients were treated with a combination of acupuncture and herbal remedies designed to improve the patient's ability to absorb and use nutrients; restore balance; unblock congested qi; and alleviate symptoms.

Table 4: Common Traditional Chinese Medicine Diagnostic Patterns In HIV/AIDS Patients with Accompanying Symptoms

DIAGNOSIS	SYMPTOMS
Spleen qi deficiency	Fatigue, lack of strength, lusterless complexion, diarrhea or thin stool, abdominal discomfort, pale tongue, and soggy pulse
Liver qi congestion	Depressed spirit, irritability or inappropriate emotions, painful distention of lateral costal region, wiry pulse
Qi deficiency	Drained white or somber white complexion, spiritual fatigue, lack of strength, spontaneous sweating, no energy to speak, low voice, poor digestion, shortness of breath, thin stool, dribbling incontinence, pale enlarged tongue, soggy pulse
Yin deficiency	Emaciation, dizziness, blurred vision, insomnia, palpitations, rising fire flush, heat in five centers, dry throat and pharynx, night sweating, seminal emission, red tongue with little or no fur, fine rapid pulse[3]

*Howard Moffett, M.S., "Using Acupuncture and Herbs for the Treatment of HIV Infection," the American College of Traditional Chinese Medicine Experience, AIDS Patient Care, August 1994, pp. 194-98.

Table 5: Comparing Symptoms at Entry and After Three Months of Treatment with Chinese Medicine*

SYMPTOM	ENTRY	THREE MONTHS
Mouth sores	39%	21%
Fatigue	94	84
Low energy	91	78
Shortness of breath	58	58
Night sweats	47	38
Low appetite	55	40
Nausea	42	40
Weight loss	46	38
Diarrhea	49	41
Lymphadenopathy (abnormal enlargement of the lymph nodes)	21	19

*Percent equals percentage of total patients with those symptoms at onset and after three months of treatment. A symptom checklist was administered to each patient monthly, and the data is self-reported, observational, and uncontrolled. In the patient symptom surveys, 28 symptoms were scored on a scale of 1-5, and according to the study data, patients reported that symptoms were reduced in both severity and number of symptoms. (Howard Moffett, M.S., "Using Acupuncture and Herbs for the Treatment of HIV Infection," American College of Traditional Chinese Medicine Experience, AIDS Patient Care, August 1994, pp.194-98.)

Studies on the Efficacy of Chinese Medicine for AIDS Treatment

According to information released by the Bastyr University AIDS Research Center in Seattle, the following research information is available about alternative therapies and AIDS.

- Howard Moffett coauthored a report in 1994 based on an uncontrolled outcomes study for HIV-positive patients. After three-month treatment courses of acupuncture and Chinese herbal therapy, the patients showed statistically decreased symptom severity and better quality of life.[3]
- In a recent San Francisco Department of Health study, findings indicate that one-third of all long-term survivors with HIV/AIDS are using Traditional Chinese Medicine. And in an ongoing San Francisco survey, 26 out of 27 long-term survivors with AIDS are reported as using Chinese medicine.

- In a study of 31 HIV-positive patients with peripheral neuropathy, results showed that acupuncture alleviated pain or tingling in 38 percent of the patients.[4]
- Lu Weibo (1994) has treated 112 HIV/AIDS patients in Tanzania with a Chinese herbal formula called Glyke, administering 60 milligrams twice a day by mouth, for three to six months. He reports improvements in CD4 counts and a reduction in symptoms.[5]

BASTYR UNIVERSITY AIDS RESEARCH CENTER IN SEATTLE, WA: NIH FUNDED PROGRAM FOR ALTERNATIVE MEDICINE RESEARCH IN HIV/AIDS

Established in 1994 through a three-year cooperative agreement with the National Institutes of Health Office of Alternative Medicine, and administered through the National Institute of Allergy and Infectious Diseases Office of AIDS, and funded with a $1 million grant, the Bastyr Center has several goals, including describing forms and patterns of use of alternative medical therapies for the treatment of HIV-positive patients, and screening and evaluating therapies for the treatment of HIV/AIDS.[6]

In late 1995 the center started establishing a network of collaborating alternative medicine clinics, with more than eighty-four alternative clinical recruitment sites joining the Bastyr practitioner network.[7] At the same time, the center began recruiting 1,500 men and women who were HIV-positive and integrating alternative medicine into their therapy as well as creating a centralized database for comparing clinical, laboratory, and quality of life outcomes for these alternative options. According to a report by the head of the center, Leanna Standish, M.D., Ph.D., primary outcome measures include progression rate of the disease, survival, changes in CD4 counts, weight, and quality of life over a two-year period. Standish reports that evidence is also being collected on whether outcomes differ in people using a combination of conventional medicine—antiviral and antibiotic prophylaxis—and alternative medicine as compared to those using either only conventional medicine or only alternative medicine. The rate of AIDS-related opportunistic infections and neoplasms in people using specific alternative modalities will be compared to the incidence of those who use only conventional medical treatments. According to Standish, the goal of this preliminary work is to sift through the treatments being used and pinpoint both the harmful and the potentially useful ones so that federal research dollars can be more effectively focused on studying treatments that are most likely to yield significant clinical trial findings.[8]

THE COMPREHENSIVE AIDS PROGRAM
IN WEST PALM BEACH, FLORIDA

Organized under the Bastyr University federal AIDS grant, the Comprehensive AIDS Program (CAP), in West Palm Beach, Florida, is one of the first sites established to participate in the nationwide study of the effectiveness of alternative therapies for AIDS patients. CAP offers acupuncture, herbs, exercise, yoga, and tai chi classes free of charge to participants. More than a hundred people are on a waiting list to receive services. And if early patient reports are any indication, these alternative treatments are working, relieving or eliminating AIDS-related symptoms. Several participants claim that the painful numbness and swelling of their feet and ankles has dissipated; stomach problems and itchy rashes are gone; their energy levels have soared; and some claim that they have regained weight that they had previously lost.

To be eligible to participate in CAP, participants must test HIV-positive, be at least eighteen years of age, and agree to use alternative therapies as part or all of their treatment regimen.[9]

Earlier Studies on ARC and AIDS

ORIENTAL MEDICAL CENTER STUDY

In 1986 the Oriental Medical Center, located in Los Angeles, studied the efficacy of Chinese herbs and acupuncture in treating AIDS Related Complex (ARC) and AIDS. After twenty months of study, the researchers, led by Jin Lin Wang, Certified Acupuncturist and M.D. (China), concluded that the use of Chinese herbs and acupuncture had positive therapeutic effects. Therapeutic treatment options were offered during the course of the treatment study.

"Acupuncture was administered once or twice weekly at the following point selections: LI4 (a large intestine acupuncture point on the metacarpus of the forefinger), which strengthens the immune system and induces the production of interferon; CV6, increases the body energy level; SP6, strengthens yin and blood; ST36, strengthens the immune system and improves

digestion; ear spleen, increases body fluids, repairs dry skin, and stimulates digestion.

Four basic herbal therapy formulas were developed for immune system strengthening which was taken orally twice each day: an antiviral formula, taken orally three times a day; a blood activator, which was given only to some patients; an anti-infection formula for high fever, which was needed for only two patients; and additional formulas were developed for specific symptoms and complications."[10]

The study produced the following findings:[11]

1. "After twenty months of clinic practitioners using Chinese herbs and acupuncture in the treatment of ARC and AIDS, the results indicate that positive therapeutic results were obtained. Laboratory results demonstrate an increase of T-4 count, and patients note a decrease in symptoms."

2. "Chinese herbs and acupuncture appear to cause no side effects. The therapeutic effect is stable, and other methods of treatment (AZT) may be used in conjunction with this program with few, if any, contraindications."

3. "None of the ARC patients progressed to AIDS. Only one of the patients had a decrease in T-cell count. This patient, however, regained normal strength and was able to return to full-time work."

4. "One patient, after starting treatment in an advanced stage of AIDS, eventually died. During treatment, his symptoms were reduced, and his pain was relieved. He lived six months longer than was anticipated during hospitalization."

5. "Although the original intention of the research was to merely relieve the immediate suffering of ARC and AIDS patients, we have found that Chinese herbs and acupuncture are well suited to treat the wide variety of symptoms manifested by this disease. We have obtained results which indicate that this method of treatment may strengthen the patient's immune system and possibly slow or stop the progression of ARC to AIDS."

THE WESTERN PHARMACOPOEIA FOR ARC AND AIDS

The financial cost of one month's supply of Western drug therapy for ARC or AIDS equals the costs of one year of acupuncture treatments.

Protease inhibitors:
Indinavir (crixivan);
Ritonavir (Norvir);
Saquinavir (Invirase);
Nelfinavir (Viracept)

The HIV virus has been shown to mutate and become resistant when patients use these drugs alone. Nausea, diarrhea, fatigue, and weight loss are the common side effects of these drugs. Cost: About $5,000 annually per drug.

Reverse transcriptase inhibitors:
Zidovudine (AZT) and Lamivudine (3TC); also known to
cause mutation and drug resistance.

Nausea, diarrhea, fatigue, and weight loss are also common side effects of these drugs. Cost: About $5,000 annually per drug.

CHINESE SNAKE GOURD STUDY

In ancient times, the Chinese snake gourd was used to induce spontaneous abortions in women. In recent years a Hong Kong scientist, Professor Yeung, has been studying the properties of this herb, because he believes it shows some potential for helping AIDS patients. Yeung discovered that properties of the snake gourd kill the trophoblast cell and also target the scavenger cells, something current AIDS drugs cannot do. Yeung, along with a research team at the Chinese University, have forwarded their findings to the United States, and snake gourd is currently under review at the FDA.[12]

Blocking Scientific Study

As the marriage between medicine in the East and West continues to meet opposition from both sides, there are those attempting to study the efficacy of herbs and acupuncture, but the answers are not coming easily. Take the case of Dr. Donald Abrams, assistant director of San Francisco General Hospital's AIDS program. According to articles in the *Sacramento Bee*, Abrams set out to determine whether varying combinations of Chinese herbs can relieve diarrhea and anemia in AIDS patients. It was his plan to study 30 patients, half of whom would get the Chinese herbs and half a placebo. Six months later, Abrams had one volunteer for the study. *Sacramento Bee* reporter Tom Philip said Abrams blames the lack of participation on several factors: the Chinese medicine practitioners were reluctant to refer patients for the study because Abrams's trial would use only one herb. Eastern practitioners never use only one herb, but rather, an individualized prescription of many herbs is developed and continually refined; the AIDS patients suffering from diarrhea didn't want to be given a placebo. Chinese medicine practitioners argued that this type of trial could not effectively measure their modalities of care.

According to the reports, Abrams modified the study after hearing the objections. Now his counterparts, a research committee at the University of California, San Francisco, rejected his new methodology, claiming it would reduce the scientific validity of his findings. Once again starting from scratch, Abrams developed a new approach and was feeling pretty good about meeting all previous objections to his trial methods. He was wrong. The Food and Drug Administration contacted the researcher and informed him that he would have to file an investigative new drug application, usually reserved for the big drug companies.

Bastyr University's Dr. Leanna Standish, among others, has called for more research on alternative therapies that show promise. Standish says that there are some promising, seemingly nontoxic therapies that deserve more rigorous evaluation in prospective controlled trials. She believes that there is justification for some percentage of NIH funding to be allocated to this heavily used yet understudied area of medicine. The question remains, however, can these alternative methods be studied in the same sterile, double-blind, placebo-controlled study formats as Western medicinal therapies?

In the meantime, people with AIDS who are using alternatives will continue to do so. The only proof they need is the fact that they are alive and their quality of life has been greatly enhanced.

> *"In 1985, my doctor told me, 'You're gonna die.' He told me to stop working out at the gym, to conserve my energy and that was it. That was eleven years ago, and I fired that doctor. I still work out at the gym, benchpressing. I've been doing everything as I've always done. You have to choose your own support and realize that the medical field very*

often is not supportive. Qigong is a way of taking charge of
your own health."

—George Wedemeyer, 55, AIDS activist

CANCER

There was Patrick, Katie, Joey, and Jose. In a matter of two months, I had written newspaper stories about each of these most incredible kids. Katie was the oldest at seventeen. Joey, the youngest, was six. And they all had cancer. Not the kind that can be zapped in a few treatments or removed in outpatient surgery. They had cancer with a capital C. The kind that people feel compelled to whisper in breathless syllables: leukemia, lymphoma. The killers.

Joey was already on his second bone marrow transplant. Patrick had been in the hospital for over a year, and after he was given megadoses of chemotherapy, the doctors felt optimistic. Katie had lost a great deal of the brain functioning that helps her remember the important things in life, such as who she is and where she put her favorite earrings. Jose, whose grandma came all the way from Argentina to support his family during his struggle with leukemia, was still waiting to see if his bone marrow transplant would take.

Touched by their determination, sincerity, and love, I marveled at their existence. Each home I entered was filled with warmth and love and that peaceful knowing that sometimes comes with difficult times. These families, no matter what the future predicted, were healed. These sick children had the ability to live happily in spite of their disease. Or perhaps it was because of their disease. I believe that these children were given a special strength, a gift of healing that comes from the unexplained, something far removed from the tubes, the chemo, the radiation. And contrary to popular medical opinion, this gift of healing is something that cannot be investigated or studied. These children knew they had been touched by something adults find hard to even consider.

I was struck with the depth and breadth of the burdens these families bore. I couldn't help but ask, Is there a better way? Is there a less invasive, less poisoning, less expensive route? A dear friend of mine, Faye Satterly, who heads up a cancer center at a community-based hospital in Charlottesville, Virginia, told me that in the past few years she too has been struck by the magnitude of the struggles to beat cancer in traditional ways. She got tired of seeing her patients get sicker and die. She got tired of thinking about the mounting costs of each chemotherapy treatment, and she decided that she had cried one too many times. With the help of her patients, she started celebrating their successes. Celebrating life, another year of survival. And at these celebrations she started giving her patients ways to improve their quality of life. She brought massage therapists into the chemotherapy area. She offered yoga classes. She purchased guided imagery tapes and Walkmans for her patients. And she started educating herself on Eastern healing and how she could integrate that into her very conventional center. Traveling to India as part of her search, she was amazed at the scene before her: the spirituality and peace of a people clearly living in poverty. On her return, she added a spiritual component to the treatment at the cancer center, and while she admits that she has not yet found the definitive answer to the most troubling dilemmas about cancer treatment and suffering, she discovered that yes, for many patients, there is a better way. A way to make living easier. A way to make dying easier. A way to make healing easier. And it is in this gentle, patient-centered way that her patients, who may still die of cancer, are healed.

An Ovarian Cancer Survivor's Story

After two bouts with cancer, thirty-two-year-old Rebecca Hotzmiller says she's not a cancer virgin anymore. Finding out that she had cancer a second time was a turning point in her life, she freely admits. And although she secretly fears that she may still die of cancer someday, she found a better way to cope with her illness. Rebecca says she has found something conventional medicine couldn't give her: hope and a chance at a future.

When her cancer returned, she talked to four different oncologists, trying to determine her best course of treatment. One said chemo. One said more surgery and chemo. One said radiation and chemo. No one could agree. That's when she decided that if these specialists couldn't get their act together and agree on what she should do, she would find her own approach to healing. And she did.

It all began when she was twenty-four, a delicate, fresh-faced woman diagnosed with ovarian cancer for the first time. Under normal circumstances, at that time in her life she might have been thinking about having babies, not destroying her chances of ever conceiving. But Rebecca had a hysterectomy, followed by extensive chemotherapy—an aspect of her cancer that she's not able to talk about comfortably. "I suffered a great loss," she says, tears brimming at the corners of her gentle eyes. "They robbed me of my right to have kids. If I had found alternative methods back then, maybe I'd have five children right now."

By the time she turned twenty-eight, the cancer had returned, and this time Rebecca lost twelve inches of her colon. Doctors said it would just be a matter of time before she would sacrifice more body parts to her disease. Some of the doctors she consulted encouraged her to go through more chemotherapy. Memories of the first course of chemo flooded her mind: she had lost thirty pounds; she was throwing up all the time; and she didn't care if she lived or died. No matter what, she says, she wasn't going to go through that again.

At first she was angry and disappointed when her cancer returned, blaming the reoccurrence on conventional Western medicine. "I had all the surgery, I had chemotherapy, and I got cancer again. I kept telling my doctors that I didn't like what was happening. I didn't want to keep losing parts of my body to this disease. But they kept disregarding my feelings, so I started reading everything I could. As far as I'm concerned, conventional medicine really failed me. I started going to a chiropractor who told me about a gynecologic acupuncturist." And that's when things started to change for Rebecca. It was at a party when the two—Rebecca and Carolyn Jaffe—actually met. Retelling her saga of chemicals and disfiguring surgeries Rebecca begged Jaffe for help. As always, Jaffe listened intently to the painful litany of Rebecca's years of suffering, and she then encouraged Rebecca to make an appointment with her.

A neophyte to the world of Eastern medicine, Rebecca wasn't exactly sure what would happen at the acupuncturist's office, but because she had done research, she knew there was hope. Rebecca believes this was when helping her body heal became a spiritual thing. Nonetheless, she was apprehensive about the acupuncture needling at first, but after her first acupuncture experience, she admits it wasn't that bad. The worst pain she says she ever felt from the hairlike needles was a sensation similar to the feeling of hitting her funny bone. And depending on which part of her body was needled, some points did not hurt at all. After extensive fine tuning of her herbal preparations, a dramatic change in her diet, regular acupuncture needling, and meditation, Rebecca remained cancer-free for over four years. On Carolyn's advice, she continued to see her Western medical doctors at the University of Pennsylvania while she was treated with acupuncture and herbal medicine (recently she switched doctors). Rebecca gets regular blood tests and CAT scans to make sure everything remains well within normal ranges.

"My doctors couldn't understand why my cancer didn't come back," she says, laughing. "I kept telling them why, but this is something they just can't explain in their terms."

—Rebecca Holzmiller

Rebecca's tumors returned this year, but she says she still feels great. It's completely different this time. There is no fear. There is no horror about the dreaded cancer. She sees conventional doctors about once a month. She gets acupuncture and herbs regularly and does everything—works, plays, lives—just like always. Rebecca feels that she is healed, even though her tumors periodically return. They get smaller. They get larger. She says that's just how it is. "My life is so different now, and my cancer does not consume my life. It's more like a part-time job. And I realize that with acupuncture and herbs, my tumors went away before, and I know that it will happen again. I just have this chronic condition."

A Word of Caution

Doctors fear that cancer patients will discard elements of Western treatment that have been proven to be effective for a particular type of cancer in favor of less invasive alternatives. Recall that although Rebecca chose to forgo her second round of chemo in favor of alternatives, she still maintained her Western medical contacts including regular testing and screening to ensure she was not getting into medical trouble. When you are pursuing any course of treatment, it is best to obtain several opinions concerning your care. As Carolyn Jaffe points out, acupuncture is not a panacea. Although it is very powerful and does cure many people, there are some who will not be helped by this type of treatment.

"We are more than just bodies. We are minds and hearts and souls."

—Breast cancer survivor

Linking Cancer and Recovery to the Mind

For thousands of years, Eastern practitioners have never wavered in their belief that healing the body depends on much more than just prescriptions for treatment. Recognizing the value of healing the mind, of having connections with the community, of finding a balance with nature, Eastern peoples have always known the richness of healing in community. And although Western medicine seems to have lost much of that connection over the past forty years, thanks in large part to the pressures of the medical industry, there are those insightful practitioners who have revived the age-old spirit of community in an attempt to improve the lives of cancer patients. The beliefs supporting the mind/body connection, however, came under incredible scrutiny when such pathfinders as Bernie Siegel, M.D., Norman Cousins, and the Simontons first presented the mind/body cancer treatment concept. But over the past two decades, mind/body techniques have become a widely discussed and often used alternative in the treatment of cancer patients.

Mind/body interventions, often designed to help patients reduce pain, control nausea and vomiting, and cope with other physical and mental disorders associated with cancer and its treatment, are helping people feel better. In addition to helping with the physical complaints associated with the disease, alternative interventions address such psychological issues as changing lifestyles, reducing stress, re-evaluating relationships, and planning for the future.[13] And as patients continue to outlive their doctor's predictions, such things as guided imagery, meditation, and support groups are becoming a regular weapon in the conventional practitioner's arsenal of treatment regimens. Nonetheless, amidst this plethora of patient tales of remission and healing, the majority of Western practitioners using alternatives do so cautiously, choosing to believe that these mind/body techniques enhance the quality of the patient's life rather than cure his or her disease. With anecdotal results far surpassing any formally conducted clinical studies on the mind/body connection to tumor regression or longevity, the medical debate will probably remain at a stalemate with most doctors viewing mind/body therapies as helpful for enhancing quality of life.

Some of California's larger health care facilities are bringing mind/body medicine into the mainstream. Kaiser Permanente—one of the largest managed care companies in the country and a willing participant in many alternative therapies—fit cancer patients with headphones and gave patients a healthy dose of guided imagery during surgery. Listening to the tape while unconscious seems to be giving patients' minds an injection of healing messages. And according to many cancer survivors who have used the technique, the tape contributed to a very quick recovery. Although many doctors can buy the fact that positive mental images can help patients improve and heal faster, and they agree that the mind and body are related,

David Spiegel, M.D., a Stanford University professor who has conducted and achieved landmark research findings in mind/body medicine and breast cancer, says we still continue to practice medicine as if the body were a headless machine in this country. Spiegel's 1989 study on women with metastatic breast cancer reported that women who took part in a support group lived an average of eighteen months longer than those who did not participate.

California Center Studies Patient Desires

Sutter Cancer Center in Sacramento, California, surveyed patients in 1994 concerning conventional and unconventional care for cancer. Nine out of ten cancer patients said that Sutter should make alternative therapies available, and nearly half of those surveyed said that they would switch their health plan to one that covered alternative care.

The Wellness Community: Patients Helping Patients

Started in 1982, the Santa Monica-based Wellness Community was one of the first and most noted programs offering psychosocial support for cancer patients. Founded by Harold Benjamin, M.D., the Wellness Community is free of charge and dedicated to helping cancer patients and their families participate actively in their fight for survival. The Wellness Community does not advocate the abandonment of traditional Western practices; all participants are informed that the program is meant to complement mainstream medical care. Because of the program's integrative philosophy, many participants are referred by their oncologists.

At the core of the Wellness Community are the basic psychosocial elements of patients supporting patients: sharing feelings; teaching self-help techniques that emphasize the idea that positive emotions and positive mental activities may improve the possibility of recovery from cancer; lectures on everything from nutrition to self-esteem; and social activities.

Bernie Siegel's Exceptional Cancer Patients Group

Even before the Wellness Community came on the alternative cancer treatment scene, internationally known surgeon and best-selling author Bernie Siegel, M.D., started his now well-known and often modeled cancer support group, Exceptional Cancer Patients (ECaP). Siegel says that his colleagues treated him as though he was crazy when he first started teaching the principles of mind/body healing. But he was determined to stand strong against the voices of scrutiny, to be a trailblazer for others. He had seen too many miracles. Too many unexplained healing phenomena. Too many times his patients proved him wrong. He'd tell a patient he or she had six months to live, and the patient would cure their cancer. He admits that he has learned much of what he teaches today from his patients. Today Siegel has finally come into his own; he is no longer that crazy man teaching his patients to visualize their cancer being destroyed or giving them a box of fat Crayolas to color with. The concepts that Siegel took such a beating for are fast becoming commonplace.

The American Cancer Society Support Programs

The American Cancer Society has played a valuable role in promoting and offering self-help, patient-to-patient programs, among them Reach to Recovery, Look Good Feel Better, and Ride to Recovery.

The ECaP program is based on the principles of *carefrontation,* a loving, safe, therapeutic confrontation that facilitates personal change and healing. Patients' dreams, drawings, and images serve as the basis for learning and awareness of the self. According to Siegel, the goal is to guide patients toward becoming exceptional cancer patients, which means people who get well unexpectedly. Although thousands of people have been drawn by Siegel's charismatic appeal, there are those cancer patients who don't approve of Siegel's tactics. They believe he makes patients feel responsible for their cancer and their healing, as if he were casting blame. Others believe that Siegel is simply teaching people how to take responsibility for their own healing.

On a personal note, my mother had a serious accident recently and broke many bones in her body. She was in excruciating pain and, when physical therapists tried to get her to walk, her legs would not leave the floor. Day after day she would walk one, maybe two steps. The pain was unbearable. I mailed her one of Siegel's healing tapes and, just before bed, she put on her Walkman and listened to his soothing words—his messages of getting your body to do what you want it to, and his healing meditations. By the end of the week she had walked over ninety steps, and she was feeling much better. I am sure there are those who will find other reasons for her dramatic progress, but I believe he helped my mother help herself.

In one of the earliest studies conducted on cancer support groups, ECaP patients fared better than cancer patients not participating in the group. The ECaP study, conducted in the early 1980s, attempted to assess the impact of the ECaP program on the survival of patients with breast cancer. Groups of eight to twelve participants met for ninety minutes once a week. Sessions included discussions of patients' problems, meditation, and mental imagery using drawings. The investigators designed a retrospective follow-up study comparing survival in a group of thirty-four ECaP participants with a group of 102 non-participants. According to reports, the study found a small increase in the length of time that some ECaP participants survived. But, as the published study reported, there were methodological failings in the study that could have affected the outcome.[14]

> *"There is no hard science answer. The people who do best are the people who say to themselves I'm going to beat this thing."*
>
> —Breast cancer survivor

Herbs and Cancer

Astragalus (*Astragalus membranaceus*)

Known in America as milk vetch, in Chinese medicine astragalus root is commonly used to treat severe qi deficiency. It builds resistance. It is often combined in prescription with ginseng, white atractylodes, *dang shen*, cinnamon, and Jujube date. In recent years astragalus has become famous for treating the side effects of Western cancer therapies. When used for such purposes, it is often prescribed in doses of about 30 grams or more a day, which is higher than the common dosage. Astragulus is sometimes used as a substitute for the more expensive ginseng.

Burdock (*Arctium lappa*)

Two studies have reported antitumor activity in animals given burdock. The National Cancer Institute has studied the herb fourteen times, with one sample showing antitumor activity in the mouse leukemia system. **Dong Quai** (*Angelica sinensis*) This versatile herb is frequently used in China for cancer treatment. In American herbalism it is used to treat several conditions including problems of the lungs and breast.

Echinacea (*Echinacea angustifolia*)
There have been more than 350 studies done on this very popular herb, also known as purple coneflower, which seems to stimulate the immune system. In laboratory tests the herb has been shown to increase the number of immune system cells (otherwise known as T cells) and developing cells in bone marrow and lymphatic tissue.

Evening Primrose Oil (*Oenothera biennis*)
Evening primrose oil can help lessen the pain of inflammation. It is especially good for ameliorating inflammation of the intestines.

Fresh Ginger and Orange Peel
Often made into a decoction for nausea.

Ginseng (*Panax ginseng*)
The revered Chinese herb, now very popular on American shores, has many uses and is often considered an all-purpose herb that can be combined with others. Some studies indicate that it enhances the immune system and reduces stress. There have been few problems reported by people taking ginseng, but it is advised that pregnant or nursing women or those with high blood pressure not take the "miracle" herb.

Mistletoe (*Viscum album*)
Both crude mistletoe and Iscador, a liquid extract from the mistletoe plant marketed by Weleda AG, Switzerland and Germany, have been studied extensively with animal subjects and have been shown to inhibit the growth of cancer cells. Mistletoe has been used to treat tumors for sixty years in other countries. The antitumor effects of this herb have been demonstrated in thirty-six studies by Helmut Kiene using people; these results are supported by studies involving animals with tumors. Other than a skin rash in some patients, there were few side effects from the treatment, as opposed to the side effects of more conventional cancer treatments, including radiation and chemotherapy. Although Weleda has a branch in the United States, it does not sell Iscador, because the product has not been approved for sale in this country.

Rehmannia (*Rehmannia glutinosa*)
Cooked Rehmannia root is often used in China to treat anemia and fatigue and to promote the healing of injured bones.

Shiitake Mushrooms (*Lentinula edodes*)
In China and Japan shiitake is known as an anticancer herb and has been shown to slow the growth of cancerous cells in animals.

Sweet Violet (*Viola odorata*)
Since 500 B.C. violets, especially the fresh leaves, have been recommended for use in a poultice to treat surface cancer.

Studies on Alternative Treatments for Cancer

All of the following studies are currently sponsored by the National Institutes of Health, Office of Alternative Medicine, except for the last one, which was carried out at Texas A&M University.

ENERGY HEALING FOR SKIN CANCER

Steve Fahrion, Ph.D., of the Menninger Clinic in Topeka, Kansas, has studied the application of energy therapy to basal cell carcinoma.

Basal cell carcinoma, which accounts for 80 percent of all non-melanoma skin cancer, is becoming increasingly common. I know several people, including my father, who were treated successfully with conventional cancer treatment for the removal of this localized lesion.

Researchers at the Menninger Clinic selected bioenergy therapy as a potential alternative to conventional treatment. Bioenergy therapy, often referred to as therapeutic touch, is practiced by specially trained healers, among them reiki masters. The practitioner places his or her hands on or near the individual being treated, the premise of the therapy being that an energy field (not necessarily electromagnetic) surrounds and is part of all living bodies, much like the Eastern concept of qi. The movement of this energy and any blockages in the energy can affect the body. The practitioner helps free the flow of that energy to promote health.

Method
The study at the Menninger Clinic involved two bioenergy healers and ten subjects found through referrals and newspaper ads. All

patients had tumors that were photographed and digitized for computer analysis; assessments were done four different times in the course of treatment. Thirty-minute treatments were given every other day for five days and involved healers moving their hands approximately one to two inches over each patient's head and body without touching the patient. Static electrical surges of up to 28 and 54 volts were measured on the bodies of the healers while they were engaged in energetic therapy. There was then one week of analysis and then a second week of treatment.

Results

Tumors were reduced or eliminated in four patients during the three-week treatment period, as confirmed by photographs. Based on the initial assessment, three of the strongest and most balanced energy fields belonged to the three participants who had the best outcomes, and the energy field with the lowest perceived strength and balance belonged to one of the patients with the worst outcome.

Most of the patients gave positive subjective reports of the treatment experience. The average cost to treat each tumor was $160.00. The researchers concluded that similar studies need to be undertaken with improved standardization of camera-client distances, the use of color film, and a longer treatment period.

USING ELECTRICITY TO ZAP CANCEROUS TUMORS

Chun-Kwang Chou City of Hope National Medical Center in Los Angeles has studied the electrochemical treatment (ECT) of tumors.

Chun-Kwang's study was conducted after significant results were achieved using electrochemical treatment for cancer by Dr. Xin Yu-ling in China. The procedure involves inserting platinum anodes into the center of a tumor and platinum cathodes into the periphery of the tumor and then maintaining a direct current between the anodes and cathodes for thirty minutes. The procedure has shown significant results in China and is currently being used in more than 500 hospitals in that country. The primary cancers treated are lung, liver, skin, and breast cancer. Chinese studies of more than 2,516 cases from 66 hospitals indicate that the ECT method has been shown very effective in treating superficial tumors and was comparable to or better than conventional surgery, radiation, or chemotherapy for treating deep tumors, not to mention that the treatment is noninvasive, simple, and economical.

Method
For the study at City of Hope National Medical Center, a team of U.S. researchers went to Beijing to witness patient treatment, and then the U.S. and Chinese scientists collaborated to obtain detailed clinical and laboratory methods and results. The study was conducted on laboratory mice and rats.

Results
In a preliminary study, treating mouse and rat tumors with proper levels of direct current, the result of treatment was long-term tumor-free survival for the rodents. According to researchers, these results are significant because rat fibrosarcoma is very difficult to cure; radiation and chemotherapy, even surgery have proven ineffective. The report concludes that more rigorous engineering and biological studies must be conducted to provide a solid foundation for recommending this promising, simple, and economical alternative method for treating localized tumors.

USING GUIDED IMAGERY TO TREAT DEPRESSION AMONG BREAST CANCER PATIENTS
Studies conducted by Patricia Newton of the Good Samaritan Hospital and Medical Center in Portland, Oregon, and Blair Justice, Ph.D., of the University of Texas, Houston, Health Science Center are among several studies that have been conducted in the past year to determine the effects of guided imagery and social support on women following breast cancer treatment. The results of Newton's and Justice's studies showed moderate changes in women's ability to cope and their level of depression. Both studies have strongly recommended further studies to determine more precisely the mind/body connection in women with breast cancer.

MASSAGE THERAPY AND REDUCING ANXIETY FOR BONE MARROW TRANSPLANT PATIENTS
Autologous bone marrow transplants are extremely unpleasant for patients because they receive high doses of chemotherapy, undergo severe immunosuppression, and they have to endure lengthy hospital stays. Tim Ahles and a team of researchers at the Dartmouth-Hitchcock Medical Center in Lebanon, New Hampshire, has studied the efficacy of massage therapy for treating the anxiety experienced by bone marrow transplant candidates.

Method

Among the patients scheduled to undergo bone marrow transplants at the medical center, some were randomly assigned to receive massage therapy, consisting of three twenty-minute sessions of shoulder, neck, head, and facial massage each week for three weeks during their hospital stay; others received standard treatment.

Results

Patients in the massage group had significantly lower scores on the anxiety inventory—distress, nausea, and lower diastolic blood pressure—as well as a trend toward lower scores for fatigue. Researchers concluded that the positive impact of massage in reducing anxiety is especially important mid-treatment, because that is the most physically and psychologically stressful part of the process for the patient. Massage is a potentially useful intervention to help patients cope with the extremely intense stress associated with bone marrow transplantation, according to the conclusions of the study.

Cancer Fighting Activities

- Make a date with yourself, mark it on your calendar and do something that you love. Perhaps something that no one else in your family likes to do, so go alone and savor every moment of it.
- Take time for yourself. Get to know who you are. What do you really like? What do you really want out of life?
- On your lunch hour, leave the building. Take a walk. Sit on a bench and enjoy the special picnic you packed for yourself. Read a good book. People watch. Write poetry. Watch the clouds transform into beautiful sky sculptures. Or do my favorite thing: daydream. I can do that for hours!
- Take a bath by candlelight.
- Go to the mountains and breathe the smells and feel nature's energy. I rarely miss a day hiking. It's my saving grace.
- Go fishing and dangle your toes in the water.
- Go to the beach.
- Window shop.
- Treat every day like it is the only one you have.
- Find a cause or shelter or something else you really believe in and volunteer your time to help others.
- Meditate every day.

- Exercise moderately several times a week. You can walk in winter, too!
- Look at your diet and consider getting rid of all that sugar or fat.
- Examine your lifestyle: Do you smoke? Are you sedentary? Are you stressed out? Discover ways to make changes in your life.
- Find what makes your heart beat passionately and pursue your passion.
- Discover your spiritual center.
- Love.

"At some point you do cross a bridge and face the seriousness of your condition. You've got it and that's OK. The important thing is to realize that this is the only day that counts, and it takes a while to come to that."

— Elizabeth Zintle, lung cancer patient

Elizabeth was the mother of one of my students who spoke to me just weeks before her death in February 1997. And even at that moment she spoke of the future. Knowing she had no cure, she was healed.

Diet and Cancer

The choices you make in your diet can be your best weapon in preventing or retarding the growth of cancer, says the National Cancer Institute, which pins the blame for nearly one-third of all cancers on diet. In recent years, the American Cancer Society has come out with dietary guidelines—recommending lowering consumption of fat, alcohol, and salt-cured and smoked foods, while increasing intake of fruits, vegetables, and whole grains—very similar to diets proposed by alternative and Eastern practitioners. Because there is a lack of systematic studies on these alternative/Eastern diets, they are open for criticism by many conventional Western practitioners, who argue that the effects of such diets cannot be judged adequately.

DR. BLOCK'S ANTICANCER DIET

One such anticancer diet was developed over the past decade by Keith I. Block, M.D., a physician who practices in Evanston, Illinois. He and other practitioners use his dietary program in conjunction with mainstream cancer care; the diet is intended to be an adjunct to care, not a substitute for conventional treatment. Under Block's treatment protocol, individualized dietary guidelines and nutritional treatments are used in combination with mainstream cancer treatment, exercise, and psychosocial support strategies for reducing stress. The patient's dietary guidelines are developed individually and based on nutritional assessments, body composition analysis, blood and laboratory studies, the nitrogen balance in the body, and other biochemical and clinical evaluations. Block says that patients are given a range of food choices from five food groups: cereals, other grains, vegetables, fruits, fats, and proteins. These groups are then divided into food exchange lists, so patients have some selection in their diet.

Block's recommended semi-vegetarian diet, which is based on macrobiotic principles, consists of high-fiber, low-fat, protein-restricted foods combined with soybean products, shiitake mushrooms, and sea vegetables. The doctor recommends that patients get 50 to 60 percent of their caloric intake from complex carbohydrates, 12 to 15 percent of calories from fat, and the remaining portion from protein sources. These numbers are often modified on an individual basis, depending on patient requirements. Pure macrobiotic diets have come under considerable medical criticism in recent years, but a nutritional analysis of Block's program indicates that his theories and recommendations are nutritionally sound. Recommended dietary (daily) allowances are met or exceeded for the majority of necessary nutrients, and the diet exceeds requirements for vitamins B, C, and B12, as well as calcium, iron, magnesium, and several other elements.

According to Block, his adjunctive dietary program has several goals, including enhancing the quality of the patient's life. Based on his observation, many of his patients are faring better on this diet and are meeting many of the goals of the program. Few of his cancer patients experience weight loss or lose their hair during chemotherapy, and he believes that the high intake of vegetables rich in vitamin A enhances the patient's response to conventional cancer treatments. According to Block and others, his program also helps to diminish the side effects of conventional treatments, thus improving the patient's quality of life. Although the efficacy of Block's diet and theories has not been clinically proven, his dietary recommendations strongly resemble traditional Asian diets and the Asian Diet Pyramid recently developed by a U.S. research team from Cornell University, Harvard School of Public Health, and Oldways Preservation and Exchange Trust (see Chapter Six).

A newly conceived research study out of the University of California, Davis, that is examining the link between diet and cancer, also has many similar food offerings: lots of vegetables, soy products, shiitake mushrooms, and grains and cereals.

STUDIES ON THE ANTICANCER PROPERTIES OF ASIAN DIETS

Although many dietary suggestions for cancer patients remain speculative, a lot of researchers are looking for anticancer effects in foods and eating patterns that parallel the Asian diet. Many have been actively following diets of Asian men and women for several years now and are starting to develop some conclusions about the effects. Examining the cancer-fighting properties in vegetables and fruits like soybeans, carrots, and tomatoes, they are theorizing about the link between the high intake of these foods and lower cancer rates among Asian peoples. There are those who are looking at the link between the diets of Asian women and a much lower rate of breast cancer (see Chapter Six, the China Project).

At the University of California, Davis, researchers are looking at diets containing such foods as tofu and lots of vegetables as potential cancer fighters. The lead investigator for this study, Mary Haan, M.D., says that previous studies have been historical reflections of a population's eating patterns. Haan is developing her own American population to track for a fifteen-year period. She is also in the process of recruiting postmenopausal women for her national effort, known as the Women's Health Initiative, which aims to track 163,000 women to determine if diet, calcium, Vitamin D, and hormone therapy might prevent heart disease and cancer. Simultaneously, Haan is recruiting 500 breast cancer survivors to determine if vegetables help prevent a recurrence of the cancer. The breast cancer study, called Women's Healthy Eating and Living (WHEL), will track women for eight years.

SOME POTENTIAL CANCER BLOCKERS

The National Cancer Institute is currently studying garlic and its cancer-blocking properties. According to a recent NCI study of 4,000 individuals with diets high in garlic and onions hailing from Italy and China, these people had a substantially lower incidence of cancer than those with diets devoid of the pungent food. The NCI also reported that in the Georgia county that grows the sweet vidalia onion, the residents have a

50 percent lower incidence of stomach cancer than do the residents of the remainder of the state, and one-third lower than the rest of the nation.

A variety of limited studies in laboratories have shown that the following foods may help block cancer in animals.

> **Teas** (green tea and oolong tea): According to researchers at Rutgers University, drinking green tea stopped 87 percent of skin cancers, 58 percent of stomach cancers, and 56 percent of lung cancers in mice;
>
> **Vegetables:** tomatoes, carrots, garlic (it is believed that in 460 B.C. Hippocrates used garlic to treat uterine cancer), onions, spinach, kale, broccoli —choose the dark green leafy veggies—cabbage, turnips, and squash;
>
> **Soybeans:** tofu, tempeh, etc.;
>
> **Shiitake mushrooms:** In China and Japan shiitake mushrooms are known as an anticancer food and have been shown to slow the growth of cancerous cells in animals;
>
> **Fruits:** especially those rich in vitamin C;
>
> **Wheat bran;**
>
> **Grains and beans;**
>
> **Licorice** (*Glycyrrhiza glabra*): A few small studies indicate that the triterpenoids in this herb can cause some precancerous conditions to reverse;
>
> **Seaweed, kelp.**

DIETARY RECOMMENDATIONS FROM
THE NATIONAL CANCER INSTITUTE

- Increase fiber in the diet: Fruits and vegetables, especially the large green leafy veggies such as spinach, beet greens, endive, romaine lettuce, escarole, and broccoli.
- Eat dried beans (legumes) and peas.
- Eat more small meals and skip the fast-food line.
- Cut down on beef and fat; only 20 percent of total calories should come from fat.
- Limit alcohol intake.
- Increase calcium in your diet.
- Increase consumption of vitamin A, which is associated with lower risk of oral, lung, and cervical cancers.

PLANTS AND FOODS CAN HELP PREVENT PROSTATE CANCER

According to researchers at Texas A&M University, a diet rich in the right foods may someday replace surgery and conventional medications to prevent and treat prostate cancer. Scientists at the university's Institute of Biosciences and Technology in Houston claim that their studies indicate that a diet rich in vegetables, fruits, whole grains, and soy products could help men avoid prostate cancer, the second leading cause of death among men.

The lead biologist on the study, Wallace McKeehan, says that prostate disease is much less common in Asia than in the West. And the university's preliminary research points to two preventative factors that can help keep prostates working properly: Eating an Asian diet and taking extracts from the saw palmetto berry (*Serenoa repens*) and the bark of the African tree (*Pygeum africanum*); both supplements can be purchased in health food stores. "American doctors have largely ignored these beneficial nutriceuticals [non-food dietary products]," says McKeehan. "But European doctors are prescribing both to prevent prostate cancer and replace surgery for prostate problems."

FIVE

The Healing Relationship

"Seventeen years ago I couldn't keep a job, food in my stomach or a home. I was angry, depressed. Therapy wasn't helping. Western medicine seemed repetitive, painful, insensitive, and useless. I consulted with an acupuncturist per her suggestion, so that my ability to live could be addressed. Everything has changed through this process, most important, my ability to care for myself as an empowered individual, not a victim!"

—Former female welfare recipient

THE HEALING ENVIRONMENT

The room is white and sterile. Everything seems tinted with subtle shades of green. Bright, shiny chrome accents the tables, tools, and glass-fronted cabinets that house all sorts of medical paraphernalia. The thermostat is set just a little too low—you're certain they've done it on purpose. As you sit on the edge of the hard examining table, the hair on your legs stands out straight, as the scent of rubbing alcohol burns the edges of your nostrils. Thoughts rush though your head, and you think that the gown you're wearing is too small. You wish you'd left your socks on because your toes feel cramped. Numb. And you know that as soon as the specialist comes into the room, the one you've been waiting to see for the past six months, you'll forget everything you wanted to ask him. The time continues to tick by; the silence is deafening. Ears ringing from the stillness, you begin thinking about your boss, who must certainly be checking her watch by now. It's been an hour and a half since you left. "Why did I make this appointment during month-end payroll?" you ask yourself, starting a litany of self-deprecating accusations. Your stomach knots. Your armpits sweat. "Dear God, where is the doctor?"

Sound familiar? Well, you're not alone. We've all, including doctors, felt some discomfort as we wait. In fact, doctors admit that the view is quite different from the patient's side of the table. You hear the long-awaited and dreaded approach, the chart being slipped out of its plastic holder on the other side of the door. The knob turns, your heart does a little flip, and in walks the doctor, often wearing a white coat with a stethoscope draped around the neck as a badge of honor and carrying a file packed with personal information about your scantily clad body. It's no wonder many of us dread the experience. We're often fearful, worried, sick, and, in an unfamiliar environment, it's painfully clear that the doctor has the upper hand.

Dr. D. Michael Baxter, the director of a family health care center in Reading, Pennsylvania, admits that the physician has more knowledge than the patient and encounters are often weighted on the side of the doctor. And until recently, neither doctor nor patient saw much wrong with the doctor being in charge. In fact, it wasn't even a generation ago that doctors were expected to make all the treatment and care decisions. Patients were expected to be passive participants in their care, they went along with that role, and that was OK. Dr. Baxter isn't the only one who thinks that the rules of the interaction need to change—that it's the responsibility of the patient to become informed, and the responsibility of the doctor to create an atmosphere of mutual trust and understanding. Sounds easy enough, but in Western medicine that change has proven to be difficult to put into practice. Many physicians are still looking to fix the body as if it were a machine, and patients want a whole-person approach: these two diametrically opposed concerns—the machine versus the heart—often lead to misunderstanding, dissatisfaction, and less than perfect outcomes.

There are those who believe that the entire healing process can be halted by the environment created or the words shared within the first few moments in the doctor's office. If the doctor breezes in, makes a few formal comments, remains standing, and looks at the chart rather than at you, a negative interaction has been set into motion. This lack of personal connection may leave you feeling unimportant and powerless. You may be afraid to ask questions, because all of a sudden, faced with this aloof, superior personage, your issues seem petty and trivial. And try as we might to follow all the recent popular advice about bringing a list of questions or demanding that the doctor give us the time we deserve, it's easier to read about than to actually do.

According to Claire Cassidy, Ph.D., a medical anthropologist, the physician-centered, authoritarian model of medicine, which has been the formative health care experience for most of us, encourages passivity in patients, and in some circumstances this mode of interaction can actually undermine the patient's willingness to follow the doctor's orders. Whether or not the doctor has excellent skills and the best intentions for the patient, the perceived meaning behind the exchange can have a profound impact on the patient's ability to get well.

> *"The placebo effect can be effective 70 percent of the time. Just having the patient feel the confidence that whatever you recommend is going to help them get well. There are these sham operations where they cut people open and did nothing, and 70 percent had an improvement in their chest pain."*
>
> —Sandra McLanahan, M.D., physician to the world-renowned healer, Reverend Sri Swami Satchidananda

HEALING AND THE PATIENT'S OUTLOOK

Two sociologists, Ellen Idler of Rutgers University and Stanislav Kasl of Yale Medical School, studied more than 2,800 men and women, examining how they perceived medical encounters and their opinions about their own health status. The results, which are consistent with other similar studies on more than 23,000 individuals, clearly pointed to the observation that the way an individual feels about his or her health is a much more predictable barometer for measuring what's going on with the individual than are lab tests, physical symptoms, or extensive exams alone. For example, individuals who said that their health was poor, even if it wasn't, were seven times more likely to die than those who viewed their situation as excellent.[1] In the same way doctors who convey an enthusiasm about the patient's prognosis or about a particular treatment are most successful at getting positive outcomes from patients.[2] In recent years this phenomenon has been referred to as the *placebo response*. Nonetheless, the incredible power of these positive placebo responses has been undervalued in American medicine. In its zeal to deliver highly specialized high-tech treatments in an era of managed care, the medical industry has devalued the doctor-patient relationship that makes such healing experiences possible.

> *"To have a successful relationship, I have to understand*
> *what the patient needs and respond to those needs. I teach*
> *residents to ask patients at the end of each visit, 'Did you*
> *get everything from this visit that you had hoped for?'"*
>
> —Peter A. Schwartz, M.D., director of the Department
> of Obstetrics and Gynecology, Reading Hospital,
> Reading, Pennsylvania

According to Cassidy, a negative healing effect can be created in fairly benign settings and circumstances: the color of the room; the wind created when the doctor breezes in; the lack of connection or touching; the impression the doctor makes that he or she doesn't really have time to listen to the patient; the doctor's lack of concern; or comments like "I don't really think this will work, but we'll give it a try." Cassidy calls this the *nocebo effect* and believes that it is harmful to patients. Once the doctor has made a negative suggestion, the patient may internalize feelings of anger or fear, putting the body into a state in which it is not open to healing. No matter how many college degrees or how much international acclaim the practitioner may have, he or she cannot heal a body that is incapable of responding. According to Bob Duggan, president of the Traditional Acupuncture Institute in Columbia, Maryland, it doesn't matter whether it is an Eastern or Western practitioner: the positive connection with the patient is the most important step toward healing.

You could have an acupuncturist and a Western doctor; if both breeze in and spend a few minutes with the patient in a very prescriptive manner, the results, from either practitioner, will probably be exactly the same. On the other hand, you could have a Western doctor who spends a lot of time with the patient and listens and asks about what is important to the patient, and that patient will get well.

Nocebo Effect: Case Study

Malia Monroe Kennedy was born on June 24, 1995. Initial tests showed a partial blockage in her right kidney. Doctors said it would either heal itself or surgery would be necessary. Every few months Malia had to endure another battery of tests, which her mother says were awful. "I will never forget the sight of Malia's eyes as they flashed at me. She was like a fawn trapped in the headlights of an oncoming car. And when the radiology technician strapped her chubby legs down to the specialized ultrasound table, I felt sick. The kind of sick when you get that hollow, aching pit in your stomach when you know you can't do anything." Johanna never let her daughter see her own fear as she cradled her trembling body in her warm arms. Johanna's husband, Kevin, paced in the back of the room. The specialist said things looked OK for now. Her kidney was still blocked but a low dose of antibiotics would keep her in good shape until her exam in six months. The family waited. Every fever, every cry in the night was a reminder. Is she in pain? Is it her kidney? What should they do? Not a day passed that Johanna and Kevin didn't pray for and worry about their growing daughter. They never missed a Sunday at church. They made amends to everyone, just to be sure. The uncertainty invaded their lives as they counted down the days to the next exam. Two days before Malia's first birthday they packed up for the long-awaited appointment, arriving twenty minutes early, just like the written instructions from the specialist's office had indicated. The waiting room was packed with parents and kids. The only seats were on the floor. Two hours later, they were still sitting on the floor. Finally they were summoned. Like good little sheep, they responded. A frazzled nurse, who never looked at them, rushed the faceless bodies along the sterile hall, accented by green-tinged florescent rays. Once in the exam room they began a litany of angry phrases. They were tired, frustrated, and concerned. A half hour passes and the white-coated physician flies in and plops himself on the exam table. "Why are you here?" He asks fliply. Johanna explains that it was on his instructions. "Oh, well, you were supposed to get an ultrasound," he responds, as if it was their fault. Leaving the room, never even looking at Malia or explaining their next step, he vanishes as quickly as he entered. Kevin was ready to leave. Johanna, near tears, said she had to stay. She had to know how her baby was doing. After some prodding from a nurse, they were whisked off for the ultrasound. The only positive part of the day. The technician was wonderful, telling the family much more than the specialist ever shared. And the technician talked to Malia and her Mom. Perhaps he had a wife and children. For a fleeting moment they said they felt human, with beating hearts. They returned to the specialist's office and waited. There were patient charts all over the desk. Patient names, social security numbers, and diagnoses were available for any inquisitive eye. The doctor—the same white-coated specialist—finally returns, carrying Malia's chart, which had mysteriously grown by several inches. He opened it and, reading the notes, he explains Malia's condition. But there was one problem. The chart he was referring to belonged to a Michael something. The doctor didn't realize it wasn't her chart, and so they told him.

In the more than four hours the family spent at this prestigious research university, the specialist never said *hello* to Malia. Never examined her. Never acknowledged that she existed. Voicing their dissatisfaction with the day, he laughed, moaning about how busy they were and that perhaps by the time they came back next year, perhaps they would have their act together. They filed a complaint against the doctor, who nearly a month later wrote a letter of apology.

PATIENT-CENTERED TREATMENT
OR PRACTITIONER-CENTERED TREATMENT?

Practitioner-centered, hierarchic, authoritarian, and reductionist approaches to medical treatment are at the center of the health care delivery system in the United States. To a great extent the assumption is that closeness will not develop between patient and doctor because in this medical model both patient and doctor are more or less interchangeable, like parts. This reductionist, two-world view compares everything: a more desirable form against a less desirable form, you are either the actor or the acted upon, the one holding all the power or the one waiting to be judged. According to Cassidy, typically the desirable form is superior, has power, and moves things, while the other is passive and is the one who is moved; for example, the doctor/patient.

With practitioner-centered treatment, the daily concerns of the patient, such as the stories the patient may be relaying to the physician, are merely shadows and have no bearing on discovering the root of the physical problem—certainly they can't point the way to knowledge in the same manner that an objective search can.[3] Where this treatment style is the norm, people who are ill become faceless objects—considered good patients only when they are compliant. If you're the one in the hospital always calling after the nurse or showing up at the nurse's station in your backless gown demanding that someone respond to your call bell, you are considered a troublemaker, and you get discussed among the staff. In an attempt to change this hierarchical view, Bernie Siegel tells patients, "When you have to go to the hospital, bring a trumpet and blow it when you want something. Bring body paint and create a message on your body to your surgeon. Make your voice heard, take back your power."

I am reminded of the suffering my mother has endured at the hands of Western practitioners who, over the years, have operated on her, given her bad advice, and treated her like a machine with broken parts. All the while she has remained the obedient, compliant patient with full trust in their directions. Growing up in an era when the doctor was a god, she always does everything the doctor tells her to do. My mother is a bright and strong woman, but she was putty in their hands—at times to her detriment. When she was in the hospital, the nurses knew she would wait, so they often didn't answer her call bell for hours. Once she was given the wrong medication, and because of a severe reaction to the medication error, she fell out of bed just one day after knee replacement surgery. They didn't find her for quite some time after the fall, yet my mother chose to do nothing for fear of negative repercussions. When I would come to visit her, I would be livid and want to go to administration, but following her wishes, I held back. I kept thinking, How much worse can it get? She was afraid it could get worse. She was at the mercy of those around her, a typical feeling of most patients.

But even my mother is changing. Her most recent hospital visit, after a very serious fall, was totally different. My parents didn't take the first doctor's advice; they got a second opinion from an osteopath. The osteopathic approach emphasizes the integration of the body's communication and regulatory mechanisms, the inherent defenses and healing powers of the body, the special role of the musculoskeletal system in relation to the organ systems, and an emphasis on health promotion as well as combatting disease. The osteopath's approach was much less invasive; he advised against surgery, and he took a much more natural approach to her treatment. In record time, my mother was walking and back doing her artwork. Had my parents not reclaimed their power, had my mother listened to the first doctor, she would now have an artificial shoulder and a metal plate with large exterior screws in her wrist. Instead she has her own shoulder, which has healed beautifully with the help of therapy, and she is again painting with her wrist sans the metal. She's talking about her qi moving, and my mother knows that with the right guidance, she can do it all. She taught herself to walk again, to drive again, to live.

In patient-centered treatment the doctor becomes your guide, the coach helping you to discover your ability to heal on your own. It is a very egalitarian, mutual encounter. You are no longer a passive participant and you bear at least part of the responsibility for your healing. Although the relationship remains a dualistic one, the dualism is complementary; you and the doctor are partners in the process.

Practitioners who believe in the patient-centered approach to healing confirm that the relationship affects treatment outcomes. In Eastern philosophies, the patient and the practitioner must both take steps toward each other to make the relationship work. It is this fluid movement of the two—each is a half of the whole; the one merges into the other half—that the Chinese summarize as yin and yang.

> *"I tell patients to pack body paint in their hospital bags and before surgery paint messages on their body to the surgeon. Bringing a trumpet and blowing it when you want something also works. Doctors have to start listening to their patients as whole human beings."*
>
> —Bernie Siegel, M.D., surgeon and author of *Love, Medicine and Miracles,* in an interview with the author.

QUACKBUSTERS

Although the general public need to be safeguarded against quacks in this day and age when there are not sufficient accreditation systems for training programs or state laws and boards of licensing for alternative practitioners, some watchdog organizations have gone a step further and come out against alternative medicine. One such group, the National Council Against Health Fraud, also known as Quackbusters, is a voluntary nonprofit health agency focusing on health misinformation, fraud, and quackery as public health problems. According to some of the organization's literature, Quackbusters warns of the seduction of psychological interventions, cautioning that, while such things may improve the patient's outlook, conventional means of treatment should not be abandoned, citing cases of patients harmed by so doing.

> *"Sound scientific methodology is universal and enduring. It may not be as emotionally satisfying as mysticism but it has proved to be infinitely better at controlling the diseases that plague humankind. Anti-science promoters are using the east-west myth to send a message that the popularity of*

alternative medicine is due to a growing disaffection with mainstream medicine with the implication that health care is too scientific and would be better if it were less so."

—William T. Jarvis, Ph.D., professor of Public Health
and Preventive Medicine, Loma Linda University,
president, National Council Against Health Fraud, Inc.

PATIENT-CENTERED INTEGRATED PRACTICES

At first blush, it's a fairly common sight; a family is waiting in the doctor's waiting room. The room is a bit old-fashioned, with fifties wallpaper and cozy flower-patterned chairs. But even the untrained eye notices pretty quickly that something is different here. There's incense burning, for one thing. But more important, the patients are being greeted with a hug or a comforting gesture. And based on what they are saying about their past experiences at Carolyn Jaffe's practice, it's as if they believe they have discovered the Holy Grail or the Fountain of Youth. More patients than Jaffe cares to think about are unable to pay for treatment. So she barters. Errands for acupuncture. A warmed apple cinnamon cake for nutritional counseling. A hug for herbs. It's a place of internal and external healing. It's a place that knows the beating of the human heart.

This place of comfort and healing is the Pennsylvania integrated practice of Carolyn Jaffe, a certified acupuncturist, who in some states can operate much like a primary care doctor, but not in Pennsylvania. Her partner, Judith Mellor, a registered nurse, nutritionist, pastoral counselor and Oriental medicine herbalist, left critical care nursing several years ago to join Jaffe on her journey toward helping others. The road hasn't always been an easy one. They continually face the challenge of paying the bills when the patients can't pay them. They face criticism from those hoping to catch them in a blunder. They face the exhaustion of helping everyone who walks through their doors. But in spite of it all, says Jaffe, they meet each patient gladly, helping men and women as they journey on unique paths. Jaffe says they have had an impact on her own journey. "I celebrate with each of them their struggles and conquests. They are my students and my teachers, and I am proud to have journeyed a small way with them."

When a patient calls for an appointment, Jaffe and Mellor do not ask what kind of insurance the patient has or who their managed care provider is: rather they ask the patient who he or she is. And before the initial visit, patients are mailed a very detailed fifteen-page questionnaire, asking everything from how they sleep; to their dreams, hopes, and losses; to their physical, psychological, and spiritual history.

For Jaffe it's very important that she know the person. The initial consultation, which costs about $125, lasts anywhere from two to three hours, and few stories are left untold. Jaffe's not afraid to admit that she integrates many elements into the healing process. "We usually talk for the first hour," Jaffe and Mellor say almost in unison. "We listen, take mental notes, and we observe." Not only does this first session give the duo an opportunity to begin to know the patient: it offers the patient a chance to unload. Sometimes Jaffe will acknowledge the patient's difficulty at this time—"I bet you are so tired," she might say, and many patients react to this by starting to cry. Someone hears them.

After the talking comes the complete physical exam. With the exception of blood pressure, weight, and perhaps some routine lab work, Jaffe's and Mellor's diagnostic tools are often foreign to those familiar with the Western treatment style. As soft music and herbal scents fill the room, Jaffe, often dressed in soft floral print blouses, begins. In an intimate gesture, she gently cradles the patient's wrist, taking the pulses. Her hands become her eyes. To the observer, it's as if the doctor and patient become one for that moment in time. What color is their tongue? Are their ears red? Do their fingernails have ridges or are they discolored? How do they hold their body? Do their feet turn in or out? It is all part of the diagnostic equation. According to Jaffe, the practice of Eastern medicine is laser exact; everything is taken into consideration.

Once a diagnosis is made, Jaffe and Mellor prepare a complete acupuncture and herbal prescription for the patient. Just as Jaffe's hands are her eyes as she feels the intricacies of the pulse, Mellor says she listens to the patient through the ears of a nurse, a counselor, a nutritionist, and an herbalist. Taking into consideration everything from the answers to the fifteen-page questionnaire to the conversation with the patient to the actual physical examination, the patient is then treated. A prescription might include everything from a suggestion that the patient get more hugs, or do something special for him- or herself; to nutritional counseling,(which Jaffe has some very strong opinions about); herbal preparations; acupuncture needling—Jaffe uses different forms, including Chinese, Japanese, French or American

Osteopathic acupuncture—depending on the patient's body type and diagnosis; spiritual counseling; and many times a recommendation that the patient visit a Western medical doctor.

Jaffe often integrates her prescriptions into the Western physician's therapies. She is willing to cross all invisible territorial boundaries to help those who come to her. And judging from her loyal following, one big reason Jaffe's patients feel better is because of the outpouring of love and support they receive each time they walk through her doors.

The Dogwood Institute

Founded in 1993, and first known as the Virginia Institute for Holistic Health, the Dogwood Institute was established to empower people toward self-healing in mind, body, and spirit. In the institute's modest space in Charlottesville, Virginia, conventional and alternative practitioners work side by side, complementing each other's knowledge and practices. On my first visit to the Dogwood Institute, I discovered that a nurse practitioner friend of mine, Cindy Janechild, was one of the original founders and was now vice president of this place of healing and hope. Janechild provides the conventional approach; others offer alternatives ranging from acupuncture, Feldenkrais, massage, nutritional counseling, and other Eastern traditions to the integrated medical practice of the institute's president, Peter Bower, M.D., trained in Western medicine and osteopathic manipulation as well as alternatives including herbalism and homeopathy. In addition to helping patients learn about their bodies and healing, the institute is committed to providing education and research in the field of integrated medicine.

Such a diverse practice faces many challenges. According to Janechild, some of the Eastern beliefs are not well received in what she calls a Bible Belt area.

> "The Dogwood Institute is struggling with obtaining
> reimbursement and referrals from doctors. One of the main
> stumbling blocks, especially here in the middle of the Bible
> Belt, is the issue of Western versus Eastern religion, which
> is really what the two types of healing boil down to. The
> institute has to think of the voice of the fundamentalists: yoga
> and meditation are the same as the devil and mind control to
> some people. So instead of a program on meditation, for
> example, the class is described as a sitting practice."
> —Cindy Janechild

And while the institute treads carefully in both worlds, the practitioner and patient community is responding to the offerings available. Recently people who are noted in their field have relocated to the area in support of the institute's evolving contribution to integrative medicine.

> *"The human anatomy is staggeringly beautiful. I am in awe of how absolutely phenomenal creation is; the majesty of creation, and not in a religious sense but as a scientist the way we are put together is so masterful. Our physiology is light years ahead of computers."*
>
> —Peter Bower, M.D., medical teaching faculty at the University of Virginia School of Medicine, and president of the Dogwood Institute

Sitting in with a Doctor of Integrative Medicine

He intimately cradles her head in his palm, as if shouldering this woman's burdens in his large hands. The sunlight streams through the half-raised white rice-paper shades that cover the glass-windowed wall. Autumn's hues mix with the filtered rays, warming the aquamarine room and creating a feeling of the natural, the serene.

Sitting at the head of his exam table, Peter Bower, M.D., has the relaxed air of one who is at peace with his work. His hands become one with his patient's neck, nestled just under her shoulder-length honey and gray-streaked hair. It is difficult to determine if he is doing much more than comforting a bruised psyche. The two talk about their kids, that week's soccer game, her blocked qi, and her trip to India. His voice is gentle, mirroring her own tones and energy.

The patient, Mary, is a French physician. She and Bower discuss her body, in her language: a little French, a little English, and some Spanish thrown in. She says she fears she has some stagnant qi. She's been waking up each morning and the area in her shoulder—the part that's been giving her pain and mobility problems—has been hot and damp. It doesn't look like Bower is doing anything you or I couldn't do, but all of a sudden Mary sends out the oola-las. "Too much?" he asks. "Oh no, never too much," she responds. Mary continues telling her stories. Bower listens. Letting her head roll slightly in its natural movements, the dance between practitioner and patient glides forward like a graceful waltz. He follows the rhythms and messages of her body. Then he says, "Ah, there it is. That's it."

As Bower, who now combines osteopathic manipulation and Eastern philosophies into his medical practice, explains, he can always feel the hysteresis—an inherent tissue motion; a lengthening—which he says feels slightly like pulling taffy. According to Bower, the working of the muscle is very similar to the science of plastics. He is stretching and reorienting. As he describes this feeling, Mary is still present, and he takes a moment to share his concern about what he refers to as New Age body workers. He says they call this feeling the energy movement or the energy cyst releasing. "But, no it's not that," he says.

Bower seems almost pained as he recalls his days working in emergency medicine. He says the majority of the patients who came in for care had what ER staffers commonly referred to as sham issues. The pain, the belly ache, the sham for what is really going on: a terrible life, homelessness, abuse. Says Bower, the issue was the whole person. The way he sees it, the people who were self-destructive, self-indulgent, had other things going on that he knew he couldn't help. If he gave them a narcotic to get them out of the ER, he was dissatisfied. If he denied narcotic treatment, he was dissatisfied. According to this gentle healer, the thoughts rushing through his head went against everything he had been taught. "They always told us that the drug seekers were just going to bleed me dry, just get them out of the ER." But one day it just hit him. This wasn't accurate. What about the guy who before he fell from the ladder was a carpenter? Before the fall he was working, bringing home food and money for his family. Now he can't work. Like many carpenters, he didn't have any insurance. So the guy feels like a failure and starts losing everything. His house. His wife. His kids. He's been drinking too much, and pretty soon he finds himself homeless. Well, Bower says, there's something wrong with a health care system that just turns its back on people like this. How can we be so cold? So cut and dry? That's when Bower decided he needed to search for something more. He says he found what is an elegant approach to healing in a blend of Western medicine, osteopathy, and a dabbling of Eastern herbal and other remedies. "The more I learn, the more stunned I am by the grandeur of it," he says, referring to osteopathic medicine, which he calls the American-made alternative medicine.

It includes all of Western medicine, but it is inclusive of a whole other realm. Some think alternative is either, or, but I use what works. Sometimes herbs can be as dangerous as drugs; we have to let the body's own natural healing systems work more efficiently. We are amazing in our recovery power, and we can't improve on our body's ability to heal. Bower believes strongly in the value of generational wisdom. "We've lost so much by not valuing the wisdom of our grandparents," he shares. "What is trendy and high-tech is important now, and we've been lured into believing that science should be totally divorced of the generational wisdom."

As he completes Mary's treatment, he suggests an injection of Traumeel, a homeopathic concoction of herbs and flowers. The two discuss the ingredients: daisy, chamomile, artica, belladonna, calendula, the list goes on and on. Mary says she only has some of the herbs at home and opts to pick up the preparation at the health food store. No injection today.

Bower's day continues. He sees Virginia, a pianist and harp player who swears by her newfound doctor. His conversation with Virginia is much different than with Mary. Bower says he learned long ago that "You have to put down your defenses and embrace the patient. If you can't do that, don't even start. You have to be open and willing to meet and accept the patient without any bias in between, and then you start."

Virginia, an attractive woman, whose nearly white hair makes her look like she might be in her sixties, has maintained her youthfulness in both gait and demeanor. She likes to talk, and Bower encourages her onto the exam table as she recounts her misery prior to finding him. She had been everywhere in search of pain relief. She says, "I was on all kinds of medications that weren't helping and I couldn't make it past 7 P.M. without going to bed. I couldn't function and I went to all kinds of specialists. Nothing helped." Virginia, like Mary, has musculoskeletal problems that affect her hands, shoulders, and the range of motion in her arms. Bower explains that through manual manipulation—which in Virginia's case has helped fluids circulate through the tissues and has created a balance between oppositional muscles—and herbal injections, on most days Virginia is pain free and able to live normally. Virginia agrees: "Now I rarely go to bed before 10 P.M. I am playing piano and am living normally."

"I have a very strong Western medical background. We were segmenting patients into little pieces, and no one was getting well. I was getting burned out after thirty-four years in critical care nursing and I turned my attention to prevention and the study of the body, mind, spirit connection. Now I

listen through the ears of a nurse, counselor, nutritionist,
and herbalist."

—Judith Mellor worked as a Western
critical care nurse for thirty-four years.
Today she is a partner in an acupuncture practice.

Patients Bare Their Souls

"All I can say is get a second opinion. My wife had a serious
fall and broke her shoulder in four places, her pelvis in three
places, and her wrist. The surgeon assigned to her case was
making preparations for extensive surgery. Something we
would not have even questioned in the past, the family was
concerned about such dramatic measures. A doctor friend,
who is an osteopathic surgeon, came in to give us a second
opinion. He told us bluntly that if it were his mother, he
would not do surgery, and if we still wanted the surgical
procedures, he would not do them. We opted for no surgery.
After several weeks of rehabilitation and physical therapy,
my wife is back to her oil painting, something that would
have not been possible following the surgery. She is doing
great. To think how close we came to having her operated
on, it scares me. In her case, the natural healing approach
was actually much better."

—Ken Pasch, 70
(This is my father speaking about my mother.)

"My hands started aching, I am a cook, and I do lots
of chopping motion. The doctor diagnosed me with carpal
tunnel, and gave me drugs, and said I needed surgery. The
drugs didn't help and I had lots of side effects, like mood
swings, depression, and nausea. It got to the point that I
couldn't do anything. I'd come home from work and prop
my hands up on pillows and cry. It was crippling. Friends
suggested I try acupuncture, and I'm afraid of needles, but
I went. The acupuncturist used a variety of techniques from
different angles; it was tailored to my needs. I am so much
better, and I will be forever grateful."

—Marcia L. Gyomber, 44

"I spent my life running to every medical doctor (M.D.s, psychologists, nutritionists, neurologists) I could find for generally feeling ill, weak, tired and scared, without ever getting significant help. I was always told there was not much wrong with me. But I began improving immediately after several acupuncture treatments. Acupuncture has helped me through another health crisis, specifically kidney stones, and also through several life crises involving my family. My general health and strength has improved, my anxiety problem is mainly gone, and I've been able to make other changes in my life, using homeopathy, herbs, and body work to improve my life. I'd say that acupuncture is the mainstay of my health maintenance and has supported the other positive changes in my life. My dependence on medical intervention has ceased, and the quality of my life has improved significantly."

—Female, 45, Baltimore

SIX

Mastering the Art of Living

*"Since I was a child, I was fascinated by the miracle
of life: one minute there are eggs in a bird's nest, and
magically a baby bird leaps up. I think most of us as
children are mystics, loving the wind blowing through
our hair and standing in absolute awe of the mystery
and majesty of everything around us."*

—Pali DeLevitt, Ph.D., University of Virginia
Medical School faculty

Ken is a fisherman, but not by trade. Nonetheless, while he was
hopping a plane here or negotiating a high-powered contract there, he
longed for the day his life would have more room for doing the things
he liked best—like fishing and more fishing. And since his retirement
a few years ago, he often keeps the same hours, leaving his York,
Pennsylvania, home long before the sun has had a chance to cast any
stray beams across his suburban macadam drive. But now he's doing
just what he wants. Rarely does he come back with any fish. And it
doesn't matter, he says. Sitting on the misty water's edge, waiting for
the nibble of the teasing fish—over time and seasons he had had his
share come to him—he danced in his mind. With himself. With
nature. It is a dance of meditation, of prayer, of peace. A dance that
Sandra McLanahan, M.D., says more of us need to learn.

"There are those who have said that illness is the Western world's
only means of meditating," says McLanahan, who is executive director
of the Integral Health Center in Buckingham, Virginia, and physician to

the world-renowned spiritual healer the Reverend Sri Swami Satchidananda. "It's the only time we give ourselves permission to stop. To take a day off from work, to do nothing."

When we give our mind the freedom to dream and our body time to rest, we start the cycle of self-repair. McLanahan says we have forgotten how to live. Convinced that learning to live with ease is the key to eliminating disease, McLanahan travels the country, and actually the globe, spreading her gospel, and many come to her center in rural Virginia for guidance.

Some of her earliest work with cardiac diet guru Dean Ornish, M.D., has transformed the lives of many people over the twenty years the two have taught and learned together. She believes that the emphasis of treatment must be on education, because doctors should be teachers. And helping patients learn the art of living is what it's all about for McLanahan. "In our culture we are very driven and very stressed," she says. Part of adjusting to wellness includes balancing our lives and learning to take time for ourselves. From this, McLanahan is convinced we will learn the importance of living a more simplified life. We rarely give ourselves permission to sit down and do nothing. It is really about the art of living and loving in a connected, compassionate, communal way with everything we do. We have to get in touch with our own inner healer: to get optimum sleep, optimum eating habits so that the digestive tract is restful, and optimum exercise so that the body can heal itself. We have to learn new skills, and sometimes we can do so only after a crisis, she says. For some, the transformation comes following the death of a friend or a child; with the onset of a life-threatening illness, like cancer or AIDS; or with loneliness. And it is in this trauma that healing begins. But why must the painful poignancy of loss act as the trigger for this change? McLanahan responds:

"Most of the people who come to me are ready for something different because they have tried what doesn't work. We don't have a health care system; we have an illness system. One thing integrative medicine can do is teach people. And that will begin to provide people with the tools for change."

McLanahan believes in the power of meditation and yoga, but she says it must be in tandem with exercise that makes you sweat. The combination of active exercise, which gets the blood flowing to the arms and legs, and relaxation training, which draws the blood supply internally, will help transform us. "I try to give my patients enthusiasm and tell them that by making such and such change they will feel the results. I encourage them to try it, see how it goes, and so often they do well," shares an impassioned McLanahan, who tries to live her own teachings. When not traveling, spends her time in a very modest white cottage tucked away in rural Virginia. From this simplified place of peace and healing that sits on the edge of the one thousand acre healing retreat known as Yogaville, a lot happens. Working with a chiropractor, an acupuncturist, a psychotherapist, and a massage therapist, McLanahan's family medical practice is thriving. People come from all over the world to seek her guidance and teachings about changing life patterns and behaviors. "What I began to see in medicine, so much of what was wrong with people has to do with lifestyle," she says, adding that Western medicine, while useful for diagnosing illness, doesn't address the root of illness. The answer isn't always found in drugs and surgery, thus Western practitioners are often left without the tools to help people heal their own bodies.

Other more gentle therapies—things that don't hurt the body but, rather, encourage the body to heal—should be the primary treatments taught in medical school, according to McLanahan. Using a combination of a low-fat, high-fiber diet, exercise, herbs, vitamins, supplements, homeopathy, and flower and gem essences, she takes an eclectic approach to healing. And McLanahan is not opposed to trying different approaches; if one thing doesn't work, she'll try another.

"That's why I work with other practitioners, I am very interested in seeing what is appropriate for each person. I do use Western medicine, sometimes, when it is appropriate. If I need to write a prescription, I do it. And I help patients get access to herbs, which most health food stores now carry. Some of the pharmacies also carry higher potency homeopathics. I prescribe based on my experience, but people can educate themselves, and lots of people are doing just that."

McLanahan says that change is upon us, and the general public will force this change. She likens this healing journey toward alternative, more patient-centered treatment to what has happened over the past twenty years with childbirth. It wasn't doctors who said, "Let's invite fathers into the delivery room. Let's make the birth experience more like home." It was the patients who were insisting on more. And as pregnant women began to demand alternatives to a negative birth experience, the market and availability of more personalized options moved to accommodate women. Now natural, family-centered birthing is available in most hospitals. McLanahan says that natural healing options will become the norm within the next five to ten years, adding that Western medicine will still have its place for some conditions, and in particular, life-threatening trauma. But, according to this doctor who lives her own medicine, we must first learn to make changes within ourselves. "That's why I love India so much," says McLanahan," they have such a strong sense of family and love. We're searching for that in this country. As Mother Teresa said, loneliness is the poverty of the West."

> "Today's medical students will be the vanguard of new
> healers . . . . they will learn that love is more important
> than knowledge, that everything is possible, and everything
> is true."
>
> —Pali DeLevitt

THE POWER OF LOVE

According to many healers, love is the most powerful healing factor of all. McLanahan cites studies that have shown that babies who are not touched die. So what happens to adults who are not loved and touched? They get sick. Says McLanahan, it's clear and simple, love can be such a powerful healer. According to McLanahan, trying to fill the emptiness, people turn to food, cigarettes, or alcohol. She believes that 80 percent of all illness is stress related, and she divides the core reasons behind disease into four categories: cigarettes, alcohol, stress, and the wrong diet. If we changed these things in our lives, we would virtually eliminate many of the diseases we face today.

> "Any path is only a path, and there is no affront to oneself
> or to others in dropping it if that is what your heart tells
> you."
>
> —Carlos Castaneda

YOGA: THE CORE OF HEALING, THE KEY TO LIFE

According to Dr. Sandra McLanahan, yoga is at the core of healing, something she discovered on her own healing journey. When she was in medical school twenty-five years ago, she was having problems with her back, and someone suggested a yoga class. "At first I thought I would have to tie myself into knots, but I discovered that it is amazingly refreshing, and it turned out to be very good for my back. I said to myself, this is very good medicine. So I have been studying the medical benefits of yoga ever since."

In her travels to India, McLanahan found many hospitals using yoga to treat their patients. "When I went to my first yoga class, I could barely touch my knees, and in a month I was touching my toes That's what happens; your flexibility returns. Any baby can do all the yoga postures like putting their toe in their mouth." There are fifteen recommended gentle postures. She continues, "This is really all about returning the circulatory competence to the body so it can do the proper repair work.

"Yoga is not a physical science but a mental science. It teaches you how to choose to be connected, and you're happy when you are connected with what you are doing. But how do you teach your mind to do that? It is a matter of training," she says. It's really like the fountain of youth. "I'm fifty, and I attribute my success to doing yoga because it really does provide the body an ability to repair itself."

McLanahan recommends exercising for one hour, three to five times per week, along with practicing yoga in the morning and meditating at night. That's the key to a healthy life, she says.

BODY/MIND CONNECTIONS

Over the years, tremendous advances in medicine and technology have contributed to increases in life expectancy rates in this country. Despite this fact, people have still wanted more in terms of healing. For many, something is missing. And recently that missing ingredient—the connection between the mind and the body—has started to find its way back into Western medical practices. It is important to note that in making mind/body references, the two are viewed as a whole, working in tandem. The mind, according to researchers, is not a separate entity acting on the body;[1] the mind and body, working together, contribute to the overall process of healing.

A growing number of medical professionals are combining technological and scientific innovation with old mind/body wisdom. According to experts in the field, with the help of these mind/body interventions, patients look at their illness in different ways, often distinguishing between healing and curing. At Harvard Medical School, the Mind/Body Medical Institute, which was founded by Herbert Benson, M.D., trains doctors in what Benson calls "remembered wellness." According to this pioneer in mind/body interventions, doctors are starting to recognize that they need to offer patients healing, not just treatments.[2] Patients around the nation have reduced their need for medications, they are recovering from surgical procedures more rapidly, their chronic pain has been reduced, and many of their medical problems have been eliminated.

Certain physical disorders such as stomach and intestinal problems, migraines, insomnia, allergies, arthritis, high blood pressure, and cancer are particularly responsive to mind/body techniques. Some patients completely eliminate their ailments; others learn how to cope with their condition and improve the quality of their life.

> *"The grand essentials to happiness in this life are something to do, something to love, and something to hope for."*
>
> —Joseph Addison

GUIDED IMAGERY

Since the earliest times, Eastern spiritual healers have used visualization or meditation to help their followers, and in recent years Western practitioners are also guiding patients toward picturing a positive healing environment. Such self-styled thinkers as Bernie Siegel, M.D., Dean Ornish, M.D., and Herbert Benson, M.D., use visualization and meditation as a means of helping patients heal. And research has shown that their methods are working. Several years ago, Shakti Gawain's *Creative Visualization* motivated the painting of mental and physical images, which helped people make changes in their bodies and external world. Rebecca, now twenty-five, says that while in high school she taught herself to play basketball and lacrosse through visualization. Although an avid field hockey player, she had never played these sports and wanted desperately to make the teams. Each day she would put a guided imagery tape in her Walkman to begin her visualization ritual. She watched as she shot hoops and scooped up the ball in her mind. Soon her images included reading her name on the list of those chosen to play. With the guided imagery, coupled with basement practice that actually put hundreds of dents in the wall, Rebecca made both teams, and at the end of the lacrosse season she was voted most improved player by her coach.

While most of us merely think of the *seeing* part of guided imagery, we often discount our other senses, which can also be effective healing tools. A few years ago, nursing homes started using aromatherapy with Alzheimer's patients. The scent of fresh basil or oregano helped people recall pieces of their life that had been buried with the progression of their disease. And numerous studies now indicate that mental imagery, whether visual, aural, tactile, or olfactory, can result in significant psychological and biochemical changes.[3] While all the reasons behind these changes remain unclear, researchers and practitioners have been able to document patient improvement and, in some cases, unexplained instances of remission of disease. Guided imagery is commonly used in the treatment of cancer patients, and studies have shown that it has helped balance and immobilize immune systems, relieve the nausea and vomiting associated with chemotherapy, and control pain.[4]

MEDITATION

The practice of relaxing the body and calming the mind came to our shores through Eastern religious practices from such countries as China, Japan, and India. Meditation is a very personal activity. It is a way of coming into contact with our own inner energy. Focusing on a candle, chanting a mantra, journeying the rosary, or staring at a mandala can help focus the mind. And there are those who claim that concentrating on a sport or martial arts like T'ai-Chi Ch'uan or aikido are also means of meditating. But no matter what works for you, studies have shown that meditation effects changes in the heart rate and respiration, which in turn reduce stress.[5] Because it promotes a sense of deep relaxation, meditation can decrease anxiety, help you achieve greater mental clarity, and improve your sense of well-being.

Although meditation has been used for deeply spiritual awakenings and creative insights, it has also been used to help with chronic pain, cancer and the side effects of treatment, headaches, asthma, insomnia, fear, high blood pressure, and heart disease.

Developed by Indian leader Maharishi Majesh Yogi, transcendental meditation(TM) is a very simple practice. You begin by sitting in a comfortable position and silently repeating a word or sound over and over again. If a thought other than the meditative word comes to mind, you repeat the word or sound again. It has been said that the level of rest achieved by TM is deeper than sleep. First gaining popularity in America in the sixties, TM was very popular among Hollywood's glitterati. In 1968 Herbert Benson, then a Harvard cardiologist, was asked to test TM practitioners to see to what extent they could lower their blood pressure.[6] After some persuading, Benson did. His studies were followed by many more, which generally determined that the use of TM is associated with decreased incidence of health care use; reduction of chronic pain; improved quality of life and increased longevity; the lowering of high blood pressure; the reduction of substance abuse; and lowered blood cholesterol levels.[7]

SEVEN

Eating Your Way to Wellness

"We have to get in touch with our inner healer: to get optimum sleep; optimum eating habits so that the digestive tract is restful; and optimum exercise so that the body can heal itself."

—Sandra McLanahan, M.D.

Nutrition has certainly taken a beating in the past few years: low-fat diets are good; too little fat is bad; decreasing protein is good; eating vegetarian is bad; eating vegetarian is good; add protein powder to every carbohydrate; eat more fiber; eat less fiber; eat more dairy to prevent osteoporosis; cut down on dairy because it's bad for choles-terol. There's a book for every diet and a diet for every illness. As the debate continues, it's pretty difficult to decide which is the best path for you and your family.

To further complicate things, because of our hurried lives, we are tempted to dine out. Unfortunately, take-out food is often laden with calories, fat, and preservatives—a tempting proposition to the palate, but deadly for one's health. Recent research indicates there may be an answer to this troubling dilemma.

THE CHINA PROJECT: ESTABLISHING A CONNECTION BETWEEN DIET AND DISEASE

It all started when two researchers—one from America, one from China —got together. Dr. Chen Junshi of the Chinese Academy of Preventive Medicine in Beijing took a year's sabbatical to work in this country with Cornell researcher Dr. T. Colin Campbell. Mutual interests and scholarly wisdom set the two on a path that created the foundations of the China Project, a living laboratory of people's eating habits, diseases, and the connection between the two in other cultures.

The China Project is one of the world's largest culturally related nutritional studies. Someday it may change the course of America's view on the connection between eating habits and disease.

In 1983 researchers from Cornell University, the Chinese Academy of Preventive Medicine, the Chinese Academy of Medical Sciences, and Oxford University in England, began to gather data on how people lived and died in sixty-five counties across the People's Republic of China. The counties were selected after the researchers had reviewed comprehensive data on death rates from specific diseases for about 80 million Chinese people; the data had been compiled by the Chinese government. The counties were chosen because of the extensive death rate data (by disease) available on the individuals who had lived there. It is interesting to note that unlike Americans who move from home to home and state to state regularly, the Chinese generally tend to stay in the same village or community for generations.

Another important control in the study was that the individuals in selected Chinese villages maintained the same dietary patterns, whereas in America we often eat a very eclectic diet—bagels and coffee for breakfast, a Greek salad and soup for lunch, and Mexican enchiladas for dinner. The stability and consistent eating habits of the Chinese made the study of certain eating patterns and their relationship to disease easier to track over longer periods of time.

By 1989 the researchers were ready to go into the field. They traveled across the rugged terrain of China's mountains and valleys to reach nomads living near the Russian border and journeyed to the far reaches of the Gobi Desert, trying to find answers to such questions as, Why did men in one part of China die of esophageal cancer 435 times more frequently than men living in another county? or Why did twenty times as many women from one county suffer from breast cancer as compared with those from another? On their pilgrimage, the researchers examined, prodded, observed, and interviewed 10,200 Chinese and

Tawanese adults and their families, collecting a thousand pieces of information.[1]

Certain patterns emerged quickly from the data. One of the first findings was that certain groups of diseases occurred in clusters where individuals had similar geographic and economic backgrounds. These ideas developed the basis for further study. Breaking diseases into two groups—diseases of affluence and diseases of poverty—the China Project researchers were able to point to information that clearly showed patterns of dietary influence on the incidence of certain diseases in the Chinese population.

China Project Disease Groupings

Diseases of Affluence: colon cancer, lung cancer, breast cancer, leukemia, diabetes, coronary disease, brain cancer, stomach cancer, and liver cancer

Diseases of Poverty: pneumonia, intestinal obstruction, peptic ulcer, digestive diseases, nephritis, pulmonary tuberculosis, non-TB infectious diseases, parasitic diseases, eclampsia, rheumatic heart disease, metabolic and endocrine diseases other than diabetes, diseases of pregnancy other than eclampsia[2]

The Price We Pay for Affluence

Prior to the release of preliminary data from the China Project in 1996, the World Health Organization in 1990 had discussed the correlation between the diets of the wealthy and the emergence of chronic, non-infectious diseases such as heart disease, cancer, diabetes, gallstones, dental cavities, and bone and joint diseases. In diseases of affluence, excesses are a contributing factor: there's too much fat, too much animal protein, too much dairy. There is no question that many Americans suffer from diseases of affluence. In fact, the focus of America's public health policy in recent years has been on finding ways to prevent disease caused by eating too much of the wrong foods. This public health issue points to a different set of nutritional problems often precipitated by eating fast food and living in a stressful environment.

In America, dietary changes come hard because powerful special interests launch multimillion dollar campaigns to make sure that their products stay on the overflowing American platter. We hear about the other white meat, the beef for dinner ads, the latest fast-food, low-fat alternative, the diet that pushes high protein, the next one that pushes no fat, then no meat, then all meat—every group has a lobby, and we are constantly bombarded with conflicting messages. In the midst of this bombardment, it is very difficult for any of us to know what the truth is.

As the China Project discovered, there are common threads linking diseases of affluence to dietary patterns; that is, people with high levels of cholesterol and urea nitrogen in the bloodstream are at higher risk for developing cancer and heart disease. (Urea nitrogen is a by-product of the body's efforts to metabolize protein.)

Interestingly, the highest cholesterol levels found in rural China were on a par with some of the lowest levels found in America; a cholesterol reading of 190 or 200 in America is fairly average, but in China it's viewed as dangerously high. Chinese women who had the highest cholesterol levels also had the highest rates of heart disease, cancer, and diabetes. Conversely, those with the lowest levels also had the lowest rates of incidence of these diseases of affluence.

What Happens When We Consume Too Much

According to the China Project research team, fat, animal protein, and meat caused people's cholesterol levels to rise. The researchers noted a correlation between high blood cholesterol levels; liver cancer, colon and rectum cancer, lung cancer, brain cancer and leukemia; and living in one of China's larger and more affluent cities like Beijing or Shanghai. They said that as affluence rose in an area, so did the consumption of animal-based protein, followed by an increase in the incidence of diseases indicative of the changed diet. Conversely, a plant-based diet made up of vegetables, fruits, and grains actually lowered blood cholesterol levels and lessened the incidence of cancer and other diseases of affluence.

Table 6: Average Cholesterol Levels in China and the United States*

	AVERAGE BLOOD CHOLESTEROL	TOTAL FAT INTAKE AS A % OF CALORIES
China	90-170	6-24
United States	170-290	30-46

*Taken from *The China Project: Keys to Better Health, Discovered In Our Living Laboratory*, by T. Colin Campbell, Ph.D., and Christine Cox, (Ithaca, NY: New Century Nutrition, 1996).

But it's not just the cholesterol that concerned the researchers. It was the combination of cholesterol and urea nitrogen that pointed to some significant disease connections. Of the people studied, it was the urea nitrogen link that really confirmed the researcher's theory that a plant-based diet is the best alternative. In their findings, there was a direct association between the presence of high levels of urea nitrogen (the stuff left over after protein is metabolized) and an intake of meat, milk, and eggs. It was this excess intake of protein from eating animal-based foods that was associated with the occurrence of many chronic, degenerative diseases. Researchers also noted that substituting low-fat animal products wasn't always a good thing; they claimed that a piece of low-fat turkey can be as bad for you as that piece of bacon you just passed up at the greasy diner the other day. According to their findings, the availability of low-fat meats can actually encourage people to consume greater amounts of animal protein, leading to increased production of urea nitrogen, which has been linked to cancer.

An increase in the consumption of animal protein was not the only potential problem they found with the widespread availability of lower-fat meats. Some poultry and dairy products have been found to contain foreign estrogens, the result of feeding practices designed to add weight to the animals. These estrogens eventually end up in our bloodstreams, and estrogen has been linked to cancer.

In China, 10 percent of all protein eaten comes from meat, and the remainder is plant based. In America, 70 percent of our daily protein intake comes from animal-based foods. At least according to preliminary data, the plant-based diet of the Chinese seems to be keeping many Chinese from suffering from all kinds of cancer and degenerative diseases.

Dietary Findings of the China Project

The Chinese consume more calories, about three hundred more each day than Americans do, yet they are generally less obese. As the consumption of animal-based proteins rises, so do levels of blood cholesterol and urea nitrogen, leading to increased incidences of the diseases of affluence.[3]

The higher the intake of foods rich in the antioxidants vitamin C and beta-carotene, the lower the incidence of cancer. Nutrients are most beneficial when obtained from whole foods rather than supplements.[4]

Although the Chinese eat almost no dairy foods and consume only low levels of calcium-rich foods, their incidence of osteoporosis is lower than that of the West. High-protein diets, especially those consisting of animal protein, actually contribute to the loss of calcium from the bones.[5]

Iron supplements are not necessary when following a plant-based diet. The study indicated that too much iron from meat sources may increase the risk of heart attack.[6]

High rates of breast cancer and high meat consumption appear to be linked. Reducing or eliminating animal protein from the diet can control genetic tendencies toward breast cancer. American women tend to have higher estrogen levels than Chinese women, something that has been linked to breast cancer.[7]

The higher the intake of fiber, the lower the rate of bowel cancer. Plant-based foods are rich in fiber; animal-based foods have no fiber. The Chinese eat about three times as much dietary fiber as Americans do.[8]

Diets rich in vegetables, especially whole grains and legumes, provide magnesium and vitamin B-6, both of which appear to reduce PMS symptoms. Researchers hypothesize that a high intake of soy products in Asia—tofu, soybean juice, and miso—may explain Asian women's easy passage through menopause.[9]

Stomach cancer in China is associated with consumption of improperly fermented foods and the overconsumption of salt.[10]

Men in China have the lowest rates of prostate cancer—1 in 100,000—than anywhere in the world. One in 10 American men will get prostate cancer. Chinese-American men living in San Francisco had a nineteen times greater rate of the incidence of prostate cancer than Chinese men living in China.[11]

HEART DISEASE

"We have to go beyond the (U.S. Dietary) guidelines, to a low-fat vegetarian diet," says Dr. Dean Ornish, director of the Preventive Medicine Research Institute at the University of California. "Animal products are the main culprit in what is killing us. We can absolutely live better lives without them."

American men and women, because of their diets, face a much greater risk of developing heart disease or of suffering a heart attack before they ever reach their long-awaited retirement. With the incidence of this life-threatening disease being much greater among people living in the West than for people living in the East, researchers have looked to the East for clues to unlock the mystery of this major killer. According to the American Heart Association 1.5 million Americans have acute heart attacks annually, which kill nearly 525,000. Nearly 3 percent of the U.S. population—7 million Americans—have clinical coronary heart disease, says the AHA.

Diet and Heart Disease

THE PRITIKIN DIET

While researchers have known for many years that diet and the risk of heart problems were connected, it wasn't until the mid-70s that Nathan Pritikin began advocating the use of exercise along with a low-fat, high-fiber diet to treat heart disease patients. Modeling his regimen on a vegetarian diet followed by people in Uganda, Pritikin, who himself had been told that he was at great risk of dying from heart disease, followed the diet for several years before founding the Pritikin Longevity Center in Santa Monica.

In a study of 21 men participating in the Pritikin twenty-six-day course, all the men reduced their cholesterol; 19 reduced triglyceride levels and 16 had a reduction in their estradiol. In addition, the effects of the Pritikin diet have been studied in connection with adult-onset diabetes and peripheral vascular disease. Studies suggest that the diet shows promise in controlling diabetes without drugs. In a University of California, Los Angeles, study, Dr. James Barnard placed 650 diabetic patients on the Pritikin exercise and diet plan, and in three weeks 76 percent of the newly diagnosed diabetics and 70 percent of the patients who were already on medication had normal blood sugar levels.

DEAN ORNISH'S LIFESTYLE HEART DIET

In the late 1980s California physician Dean Ornish had beliefs similar to Pritikin's; and he was able to actually demonstrate that the type of diet and exercise program Pritikin was suggesting would work. Taking before and after pictures of people's clogged blood vessels, using an angiogram, Dr. Ornish was able to actually see the effects that lifestyle and diet changes made in his patients. Based on a predominantly vegetarian diet, the Ornish plan, now called the Lifestyle

Heart Diet, allows no meat, poultry, or fish and requires that 75 percent of a person's daily calories come from carbohydrates, and less than 10 percent come from fat. Interestingly, the components of the Ornish diet are very similar to common Asian diets.

Following several previous studies of Ornish's diet, a randomized controlled trial was conducted over a period of one year. All of 28 men and women involved in this trial had partially blocked arteries and were placed on the Ornish program without the assistance of lipid-lowering drugs. Another group of 20 subjects were placed in a control group receiving conventional care. At the end of the yearlong trial the study produced the following results:

In the group on the Ornish program there was a 91 percent reduction in the frequency of angina and a 28 percent reduction in the severity of angina.

In the control group on conventional therapy there was a 165 percent increase in the frequency of angina, a 95 percent increase in the duration of angina, and a 39 percent rise in the severity of angina.

THE ASIAN DIET PYRAMID

An offshoot of the China Project, the Asian Diet Pyramid was developed as a healthful alternative to the U.S. Food Guide Pyramid, which lumps animal and plant foods together, a practice that the China Project researchers do not agree with. The China Project team of researchers linked up with Harvard University researchers and the nonprofit foundation Oldways Preservation Trust to develop the Asian Diet Pyramid unveiled at the International Conference on the Diets of Asia in late 1995. According to Dr. Campbell, the China Project's principal investigator, this pyramid has tremendous public health implications and reflects the growing body of research suggesting that Americans will not reduce their rate of cancer and heart disease until they shift their diets from animal-based foods to plant-based foods.

The Asian Diet Pyramid emphasizes a nutritional base of rice, rice products, noodles, breads, and grains, preferably whole grains and minimally processed foods. The next segment on the pyramid includes fruits, vegetables, legumes, nuts, and seeds, combined with daily physical exercise, a small amount of vegetable oil, and a moderate consumption of plant-based beverages including tea (black or green), sake, beer, and wine. A typical meal might be a heaping serving of rice surrounded by vegetables and perhaps a little tofu, tempeh or miso, with fruit for dessert. National Cancer Institute studies have discovered that the isoflavones in soy products are powerful cancer fighters. Contrary to other vegetarian diets, the Asian Pyramid Diet allows for optional choices of small daily servings of low-fat dairy products or fish; weekly servings of eggs or poultry; and monthly servings of red meat.

If you look at the Asian Diet Pyramid and wonder about things like calcium and osteoporosis, Dr. Campbell says that the minimal intake of dairy products and plant-based selections seen in the Asian diet actually correlated to a lower incidence of osteoporosis: "Western countries, with their calcium largely taken in the form of dairy products, have significantly higher rates of osteoporosis."

> *"I hope that the pyramid will point the way to additional alternatives to our traditional American diets that are high in saturated fat, trans-fatty acids, and cholesterol. It's clear that there are other ways of eating, besides the American classic of roast beef, mashed potatoes and gravy, that are both much healthier and tastier."*
>
> —Walter Willett, M.D., professor and chairman
> of the Department of Nutrition,
> Harvard School of Public Health

Released by the U.S. Department of Agriculture in 1992 to replace the older basic four food groups, the U.S. Food Guide Pyramid is designed to give Americans information on eating a balanced diet. Similar to the Asian Pyramid, fruits, vegetables, breads, grains, cereals, rice, and pasta form the base of the pyramid.

Table 7: Eastern and Western Diets: A Comparative View*

	China	America
Calories	2,636	2,360
Calcium (milligrams/day)	544	1,143
Iron (milligrams/day)	34	18
Vitamin C (milligrams/day)	140	73
Total Protein (grams/day)	64	91
Plant Protein (grams/day)	60	27
Dietary Fiber (grams/day)	33	10
Starch (grams/day)	371	120

Source: *From *The China Project: Keys to Better Health, Discovered in Our Living Laboratory,* by T. Colin Campbell, Ph.D., and Christine Cox, (Ithaca, NY: New Century Nutrition, 1996).

HEALTHFUL PROPERTIES OF FOODS

Calcium-enhancing foods other than dairy products: broccoli, tofu, soybeans, pinto beans, chickpeas, okra, kale, dried figs, raisins, dates, white beans, pineapple, and pineapple juice

Foods high in antioxidants like beta-carotene or vitamin C (look for the vibrant colors of orange and green): apricots, peaches, sweet potatoes, carrots, collard greens, kale, raw spinach, winter squash, mango, broccoli, pumpkin, sweet red or green peppers, kale, orange, grapefruit, tomatoes, papaya, and peas

Cholesterol Busters: kelp (seaweed), rice bran, green tea, garlic, onions, shiitake mushrooms, beans, soybeans, legumes, apples, carrots, and oats

Whole Foods or Supplements?

According to several studies, nutritional supplements cannot give you the same protection from disease as whole foods because whole foods have phytochemicals—indoles, phenols, and flavinoids—which work together. When one of these phytochemicals is missing, the desired effect (often minimizing the effect of free radicals that age our body's organs) cannot be achieved. Supplements do not have any phytochemicals.[12]

RDA's Weren't Intended for Consumers

The United States has been developing and regulating nutritional guidelines for more than a hundred years. Back in the earlier days nutritionists faced the challenge of how to correct nutritional deficiencies. Today, with so many excesses in our country, the dilemma is reversed, and establishing guidelines is becoming increasingly difficult. Nonetheless, about twenty years ago the U.S. Department of Agriculture developed what we now know as the recommended daily allowances (RDAs) for essential nutrients. Initially these guidelines weren't developed to help consumers to make food buying decisions; they were intended to serve as standards for planning food supplies for population groups. But today with stricter guidelines on packaging and labeling, consumers are able to use the information provided to better plan their own diets.

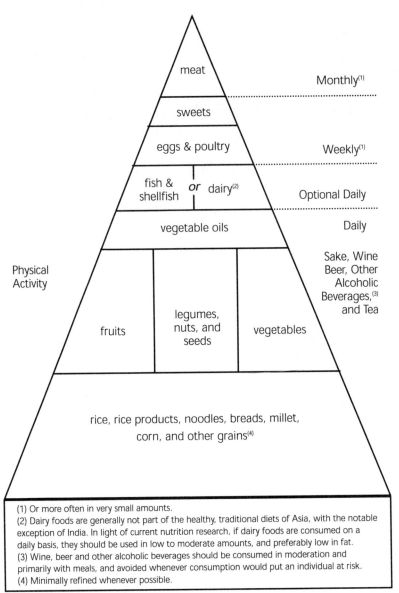

meat — Monthly[1]

sweets

eggs & poultry — Weekly[1]

fish & shellfish *or* dairy[2] — Optional Daily

vegetable oils — Daily

Physical Activity

fruits

legumes, nuts, and seeds

vegetables

Sake, Wine Beer, Other Alcoholic Beverages,[3] and Tea

rice, rice products, noodles, breads, millet, corn, and other grains[4]

(1) Or more often in very small amounts.
(2) Dairy foods are generally not part of the healthy, traditional diets of Asia, with the notable exception of India. In light of current nutrition research, if dairy foods are consumed on a daily basis, they should be used in low to moderate amounts, and preferably low in fat.
(3) Wine, beer and other alcoholic beverages should be consumed in moderation and primarily with meals, and avoided whenever consumption would put an individual at risk.
(4) Minimally refined whenever possible.

© 1995 Oldways Preservation & Exchange Trust

ASIAN DIET PYRAMID

EIGHT

Herbs: Ancient Remedies, Modern Healing

*"Following surgery this past spring I was so nauseated,
I couldn't eat. I had lost fifteen pounds, and I don't think
my doctors paid much attention to me. I couldn't even
drink water. So my massage therapist suggested I go to
this woman who sells herbs. She sold me ginger capsules,
and within a couple of weeks I was eating everything I
could before the surgery. I call it my ginger cure."*

—Marion Stapleton, Indiana

Since the earliest civilizations, humans have been on a quest to discover
the healing properties of plants. There is evidence that nearly sixty-
thousand years ago Neanderthal man discovered botanical remedies
that are still in use today. Well into this century the majority of medicines used in the Western and Eastern worlds by the neighbor up the
road or the country doctor came from plant extracts and herbal lore.
For hundreds of years it was common practice for the family doctor to
use herbs and cultural remedies in treating the sick. Our grandmothers
and great-grandmothers knew all about the healing properties of plants,
often creating gorgeous medicinal gardens. Herbs were an important
part of everyday life. Earlier in this century, prescription drugs were
most often reserved for the acutely ill, and even then a combination of
folk remedies and chemical compounds were most often used to nurse
people back to health.

Up until the 1940s pharmacology texts contained information on
the healing properties of twigs, bark, roots, berries, and flowers. It
wasn't until technology skyrocketed that we began losing touch with
our herbal heritage in this country. As we moved away from this most

valuable knowledge, regulatory bodies such as the FDA developed information strategies that portrayed herbal medicinals as worthless and potentially dangerous. This image is set in the minds of America's regulatory bureaucrats today, but the general consumer is beginning to discover the healing properties of plants and reclaiming the generational wisdom of those who went before us.

THE INCREASING POPULARITY OF HERBAL REMEDIES

The FDA might be keeping a tight lid on the use of herbal medicinals in mainstream medicine in this country, but consumers are finding a way around the limitations. In recent years the sale of herbs has increased dramatically. In 1990 about 3 percent of Americans purchased herbs for medicinal purposes. By 1994 that figure had jumped to 17 percent, says a Gallup survey. According to estimates by the American Botanical Council, sales in 1995 jumped 25 percent over sales in 1994, totaling nearly $2 billion.

REGULATORY LOCK-OUT: FDA AND HERBS IN AMERICA

Under the current FDA regulations it is very difficult for herbal remedies to be studied or prescribed in the United States. Health food stores can sell herbs and herbal preparations as dietary supplements, but the packaging cannot indicate health or medicinal uses of the herb or the FDA will remove the product from the store's shelves. This makes it very difficult for consumers and perpetuates the cycle of rising medical costs. Another reason why it is difficult for consumers to have access to herbs is because herbalists cannot be certified to practice in most states. Unless practicing with a homeopathic doctor, naturopath, or acupuncturist, it is illegal in most areas of America for an herbalist to prescribe remedies to others.

According to current FDA codes, any preparation, whether a chemical compound or an herbal remedy, must undergo the same rigorous clinical trial testing as any pharmaceutical drug. The problem is that the best therapeutic results from herbal remedies are often obtained by using a number of herbs in combination, but the FDA testing protocol requires testing one ingredient only, often isolating a particular chemical constituent of an herb. Typically concentrating on that one constituent for testing on lab animals or humans, the FDA's research does not take into account the balance of chemical constituents that make up the herb, and it can distort the reputed properties and actions of an herb.

A 1993 *Wall Street Journal* article stated that bringing a new drug into the pharmaceutical arena costs approximately $140 million to $500 million. Herbalists and university researchers cannot possibly hope to raise such sums. What is more, U.S. drug companies are not very interested in pursuing herbs and herbal formulas because botanicals cannot be patented. A manufacturer of herbal preparations could never recover the exorbitant costs of bringing its products to market under FDA criteria.

Currently the bulk of the research on botanical remedies is being conducted in Europe and Asia. Although these countries have made rapid progress in discovering herbs or, as they call them, *phytomedicines,* for treating life-threatening conditions, the U.S. research effort has declined.

Interestingly, recent studies conducted in Europe and Asia show that the effectiveness of many botanical remedies meet Western pharmaceutical clinical standards, yet the United States will not recognize the value of these herbal preparations in treating our ill and dying. Many believe that using plant-based medicinals in this country would improve public health, lower health care costs, and lead this country in the direction of prevention rather than sick care. But the current regulatory policies in the United States prevent any of these benefits from being realized. The FDA has approved a few herbal preparations for use in end-of-life heroics, but the agency has never approved the use of herbs for preventive care. Some proponents of changing the current regulatory lock-out argue that the FDA should adopt a system similar to the European system for phytomedicines. Under European regulations there is a three-tiered system in which herbal medicinals are categorized by level of toxicity, and not all are subject to such rigid standards. Herbal products, under this system, are labeled with information on the traditional uses of a given plant, and consumers are free to make informed choices about herbs.

Ancient Remedies and Modern Drugs Working Together?

In recent years a few of the drug companies, such as Merck, Interneuron Pharmaceuticals, and Rorer, have taken ancient Chinese wisdom about herbs and medicinals and have created several new drugs that are currently under clinical trial. Among the herbs they have explored are Paluther, a synthetic form of artemisinin, which has been used by the

Chinese for centuries in the treatment of malaria; and Hyperzine A, an alkaloid from the leaves of the Chinese herb tacrine, which is being studied for use with Alzheimer's patients.

The Risk of Losing the Healers, the Flora and the Fauna

There is a growing concern that as rainforests and natural areas are bulldozed to make way for more condos and shopping malls, the natural habitat for many of the plant-based medicinals will be lost forever. According to several studies, in the United States alone nearly 10 percent of all flower species will be gone by the year 2000.[1]

Just like the plants, the knowledge of ancient healers will also become extinct if we do not begin to honor the traditions of healers around the world. Few younger people are interested in taking the torch from the older generation, so the wisdom will be lost if we do not record from oral history and other sources what is known about natural forms of healing.

EASTERN AND WESTERN HERBAL TRADITIONS

Chinese herbalism dates back thousands of years and is the world's oldest continually practiced form of medicine. The Chinese are one of the only cultures that has progressively studied and added to its *materia medica* (a collection of descriptions of herbal and other preparations used to treat illness), which now has over 5,767 entries. Although acupuncture has gained interest in the United States, Chinese herbal medicine is still used mainly in China.

According to Paul Olko, a certified Chinese herbalist, the combination of herbs and Chinese massage are often medical paths reserved for the more wealthy in China, with acupuncture being used to treat many in rural villages. Unlike Western herbology, which often treats symptoms, Chinese herbalists treat imbalances in the body, such as too much wind or too much heat. A Chinese herbal prescription is based on an in-depth examination of the patient, with the practitioner taking into account the patient's physical and emotional condition. Once the practitioner determines the root of the problem, he or she develops an elaborate prescription. Olko says that some prescriptions could contain as many as fourteen ingredients, and these are often adjusted in the first few weeks to make certain that the formula is right for the patient. It is the goal of herbal medicine practitioners to eliminate side effects; so often a slight change in the combination and amounts of herbs used will take care of the problem.

In Western herbology, which dates back before Hippocrates, herbs are categorized by their actions and properties; how they work on certain ailments or interact with different parts of the body. In Chinese medicine, herbs are categorized by their relationship to the five elemental energies.

It's important to note that Chinese or Western herbal medicine doesn't mean that Chinese herbalists use only Chinese herbs or vice versa. And many times herbalists use herbs grown from around the world. The herbalist is not concerned about geographical origins of the plant, but, rather, the philosophy of herb use. Chinese herbologists feel that the best effects are still achieved from making an infusion or a decoction. Often made from woody stems, bark and seeds, the herbs are boiled in water for 15 minutes, strained, and drank hot—or tea from the herbal formula is used rather than prescribing a pill. This allows the practitioner more flexibility in adjusting the preparation, and, according to Olko, for many making the tea each day becomes part of a ritual.

Training Assures Your Safety

While some self-taught herbalists are very good, it is hard for us to know who is good and who is not. Since the wrong combinations of herbs can be toxic, it may be wise to look for a certified herbalist or a licensed acupuncturist (or other licensed alternative practitioner) to help you as you start on your herbal journey. In the United States there are several accreditation processes for herbalists. In California, acupuncturists must also pass the Chinese herbal medicine segment for licensing. The National Commission for the Certification of Acupuncturists has also created a certification process for Chinese herbal medicine, so after a certified practitioner's name there should be the letters Dipl.C.H. or Diplomate of Chinese Herbs. To be safe, ask about an herbalist's credentials before following his or her advice.

TREATING COMMON AILMENTS WITH HERBS

Over the years, while rarely recognized in America, herbs from China, India, Germany, America, and Native American traditions have been researched extensively in China, Korea, Japan, Russia, and Germany, with methods that meet even stringent Western clinical standards. Following are listings of herbs and their potential uses categorized under the ailments that they have been shown to treat based on many studies.

Addictions

Lobelia (Lobelia cardinalis)
Known as cardinal flower, lobelia was used for years to treat stomachache and syphilis. Today this herb is used for asthma and as an expectorant for bronchitis. It is said that Native Americans smoked lobelia inflata to break the nicotine addiction.

Milk Thistle (Silybum marianum)
Milk thistle has been used for centuries as a liver tonic. Studies conducted in the 1970s indicated that seed extracts helped regenerate liver cells damaged by alcohol and other drugs. Milk thistle protects the liver from toxin damage.

Sleep Tea

The Lincoln Hospital in New York City developed a combination of herbs, called Sleep Tea, to help people who are withdrawing from drugs to sleep. The mixture contains chamomile, peppermint, catnip, skullcap, hops, and yarrow. The tea, according to Dr. Michael O. Smith, the center's director, is used to promote relaxation and to treat insomnia. It is also effective in aiding alcohol detoxification if taken hourly. According to Dr. Smith, these herbs are not habit forming and do not carry a risk from overdose or misuse.

Aging

Fo-Ti/Ho shou wu (Polygonum multiflorum)
Used as a rejuvenating tonic in China, Fo-Ti is said to prevent hair from turning gray and helps people maintain strength and vitality as they age.

Ginkgo (Ginkgo biloba)
By promoting the flow of blood to the brain, ginkgo helps increase mental clarity and memory. In a French study, the efficacy of this Oriental herb for treating disorders of the brain due to aging

was found to be promising. Another study showed that ginkgo improved mobility, communication, short-term memory, and orientation. Among those who took gingko regularly, those previously unable to walk because of pain were able to do so, and some increased the distances they could walk pain-free by 30–100 percent. Circulation was also greatly enhanced.

Appetite Control

Cayenne (*Capsicum frutescens*)
Cayenne mixed into a cup of boiling water twice a day helps stimulate the appetite. Cayenne does irritate the stomach and kidneys if overused.

Guayusa (*Ilex guayusa*)
Animal studies have shown that an herbal preparation made from the leaves of this plant reduces uncontrolled appetite considerably.

Asthma

Baical Skullcap/Huang qin (*Scutellaria baicalensis*)
In laboratory studies of guinea pigs, baical skullcap root has been shown to be effective in treating allergic asthma.

Ginseng/Ren sheng (*Panax ginseng*)
First used more than three thousand years ago by the Chinese, ginseng has been called the miracle herb. There have been more than three hundred original papers published on this versatile herb. The French started using it for asthma many years ago, and it is often used as an overall tonic for the entire body.

Lobelia (*Lobelia cardinalis*)
Known as cardinal flower, this herb was used for years to treat stomachache and syphilis. Today it is used for asthma and as an expectorant for bronchitis. It is said that Native Americans smoked lobelia inflata to break the nicotine addiction.

Parsley (*Petroselinum sativum*)
Although the effects of parsley have not undergone rigid laboratory studies, our grandmothers and great-grandmothers often used parsley as an expectorant for coughs and asthma. Steep leaves in

parsley juice or oil should not be used by pregnant women.

Poke Root (*Phytolacca americana*)

A robust perennial herb that is indigenous to the eastern United
States, poke root is used to treat asthma, boils, intestinal
worms, cramps, and stomach ulcers. The herb is said to be
effective in treating parasites in both animals and humans.

Cancer

See Chapter Four, "Herbs and Cancer," for herbs that have been
researched for their efficacy in treating or helping with the side effects
of cancer.

Colds and Upper Respiratory Infections

Echinacea/Purple Coneflower (*Echinacea angustifolia*)

Native Americans introduced this herb as a snakebite potion.
One of the most highly researched herbs, echinacea is now very
popular because of its immune-enhancing properties. European
studies indicate that echinacea is very effective in treating colds,
flu, and candida.

Ephedra/Ma huang (*Ephedra sinica*)

Traditionally used by the Chinese to treat asthma, this herb acts
as a stimulant and should be avoided by people with high blood
pressure. Ma huang is found in many natural cold remedies, but
compounds derived from this herb are also found in over-the-
counter cold and allergy medications.

Eucalyptus (*Eucalyptus globulus*)

The oil of this plant has been used for many things. For years it
has been placed in steam to relieve the effects of cold and flu. It is
found in over-the-counter cough drops. When rubbed on the skin,
eucalyptus oil provides some pain relief from arthritis. It should
not be taken internally.

Fenugreek (*Trigonella graecum*)

Dating back to Hippocrates, fenugreek is a very popular folk
remedy for colds and sore throats. In a study conducted in India,
the pulverized seeds of this herb were shown to reduce blood
sugar in insulin-dependent individuals.

Lobelia (*Lobelia cardinalis*)
Known as cardinal flower, it was used for years to treat stomach-ache and syphilis. Today it is used for asthma and as an expectorant for bronchitis. It is said that Native Americans smoked lobelia inflata to break the nicotine addiction.

Pueraria/Ko Ken (*Pueraria lobata*)
Pueraria has been used by Chinese practitioners to treat flu, colds, and gastrointestinal conditions.

Rabbit Tobacco (*Gnaphalium obtusifolium*)
Originally used by the Lumbee Indians, rabbit tobacco is said to cause profuse sweating. This herb is a native plant of the eastern United States and is used to treat colds, flu, neuritis, asthma, coughs, and pneumonia.

Sweet Flag (*Acorus Calamus*)
This root has been used to treat gas, colds, coughs, sore throats, and headache. Early Native American tribes thought that sweet flag was a panacea for most ailments.

Wild Chrysanthemum Flower/ye ju hua (*Chrysanthemum indicum*) Also used to treat high blood pressure, this herb has proved effective in treating colds and bronchitis. In one study of 1,000 individuals, wild chrysanthemum flower was made into a tea and administered to people in five groups. Depending on the group—there were those who rarely got colds, those with occasional colds, and those with frequent colds—the herb was taken once a month, twice a month, or every week. When compared to the past history of those participating in the study, the incidence of colds decreased by nearly 14 percent. Simultaneously another study examined 119 cases of chronic bronchitis. Using the same preparation as was used in the cold study, researchers found that this group had a 38 percent reduction in attacks as compared with the previous year.[2]

Constipation

Cascara Sagrada (*Rhamnus purshiana*)
Also known as buckthorn, this herb is a natural laxative. It stimulates the lining of the upper intestines and promotes improved bowel function. Cascara sagrada can be purchased in capsule

form, but you should not exceed the suggested dose of 1–3 capsules daily, as overuse can cause diarrhea.

Licorice/Gan Cao *(Glycyrrhiza uralensis)*
In addition to reducing fever and inflammation, this ancient herb has many uses including relieving constipation, lowering cholesterol, and soothing sore throats and coughs.

Papaya/Fan mu gua (*Carica papaya*)
This herb has been used for centuries to treat stomachaches, indigestion, and constipation.

Psyllium (*Plantago psyllium*)
Now seen as a cholesterol buster that helps you raise high-density lipoproteins or (HDLs), psyllium has been used for centuries to treat constipation. Because of its high fiber quality, it is best to add this herb to your diet gradually to avoid gas and stomach cramping.

Diarrhea, the Flu, and Gastrointestinal Problems

Baical Skullcap/Guang qin (*Scutelleria baicalensis*)
Studies have shown that this herb inhibits the effects of bacteria. In one such study, 100 patients with dysentery received an herbal prescription with huang qin as the primary ingredient. The average recovery time was 2.5 days and a negative stool sample occurred in 4.3 days.[3]

Catnip (*Nepeta cataria*)
Catnip can ease the cramping of diarrhea.

Coptis or yellow links/Huang lian (*Coptis sinensis*)
Studies have shown that this herb is more effective than sulfa drugs in fighting certain bacteria that cause dysentery. It has also been shown to be effective against some antibiotic-resistant bacteria. In laboratory studies conducted on chicken embryos, the herb was demonstrated to be effective against the flu. Huang lian has been used to treat scarlet fever and has been shown to be as effective as penicillin or a combination of penicillin and sulfa for treating bacterial infections.

Dryopteris/Guan zhong (*Dryopteris crassirhizoma*)
Recently Guan zhong has been prescribed much like a flu vaccine, as a preventive for influenza. Clinical trials have shown that this herb can be very effective in inhibiting the flu virus.[4]

Peppermint (*Mentha piperita*)
Peppermint tea is one of the most commonly used and preferred home remedies for stomachache, but peppermint is also used for the nausea commonly experienced by migraine sufferers.

Poke Weed (*Phytolacca americana*)
A robust perennial herb that is indigenous to the eastern United States, poke weed is used to treat asthma, boils, intestinal worms, cramps, and stomach ulcers. Listed in the British Herbal Pharmacopeia, it is said to be effective in the treatment of parasites in both animals and humans.

Pueraria/Ko Ken (*Pueraria lobata*)
This herb has been used by Chinese practitioners to treat flu, colds, and gastrointestinal conditions.

Raspberry (*Rubus idaeus*)
Made into a tea, raspberry leaves can aid diarrhea cramping.

Sassafras (*Sassafras albidum*)
Common to woodland borders and aging fields, this deciduous plant is native to the northeastern United States. Sassafras is used to treat measles, chicken pox, colds, flu, and fever.

Gynecological Problems

See Chapter Nine for herbs that have been researched for their efficacy in treating or helping obstetrical and gynecological problems.

High Blood Pressure

Garlic (*Allium sativum*)
Stir-frying, which makes it more palatable for some, and eating two to three cloves of garlic a day can help lower blood pressure. Some experts argue that eating *raw* garlic is more effective.

Wild Chrysanthemum Flower/ye ju hua
(*Chrysanthemum indicum*)

Although used to treat colds and bronchitis, this herb has also been effective in lowering blood pressure. Chrysanthemum flower has been used singly or in a decoction (a tea) with jin yin hua and pu gong ying. Studies indicate that given by injection or taken orally, ye ju hua lowers blood pressure. The studies also noted that preparations using the whole plant show more toxicity and are less effective than preparations made from the flower.

Pain Relief—Headache and PMS

Corydalis Rhizone/ Yan hu suo (*Corydalis yanhusuo*)
Said to have 1 percent the strength of opium, this herb has been widely used to relieve pain, and recent studies have shown it to be effective for treating menstrual cramps.

Feverfew (*Chrysanthemum parthenium*)
This ancient herb was lost or forgotten until the late 1970s when its use was revived in Britain for treating migraines. In 1985 reports surfaced saying that feverfew extracts inhibited the release of the two substances—serotonin and prostaglandin—thought to be responsible for the onset of migraines. Taking feverfew can reduce the number of migraines and may also lessen the severity of migraine symptoms.

Peppermint (*Mentha piperita*)
Peppermint tea is one of the most commonly used and preferred home remedies for stomachache; it is also used for the nausea commonly experienced by migraine sufferers.

White willow (*Salix alba*)
Historically used for fevers, arthritis, and headaches, the bark of this tree is used like aspirin without aspirin's side effects.

Tips for Common Maladies

Try valerian for insomnia.

A tincture of cayenne may help toothaches.

Garlic or ginger cooked into foods will help eliminate gas.

A tea made of yarrow, lemon balm, mint, and elder flowers can help when you feel a cold coming on.

Goldenseal and echinacea may help relieve a bladder infection.

Try using white willow instead of aspirin.

Reduce migraines by taking feverfew daily.

If you've been overindulging, fennel suppresses appetite and relieves gas.

To clear those cobwebs out of your head, try some cinnamon.

A tea of chamomile or catnip can help relax and soothe the mind.

Butcher's Broom can help relieve bloating; it's a good diuretic.

NINE

Women and Healing: Reclaiming our Natural Processes

"Many wonderful women have had an impact on my journey. I celebrate along with each of them, their struggles and their conquests. They are my students and my teachers and I am proud to have journeyed a small way with each of them."

—Carolyn Jaffe, acupuncturist

For centuries women's health care has been in the hands of men. Although women have the natural ability to heal—the home, children, the earth—women, until recently, have been prohibited from participating in healing rituals. And since the earliest of times in our Western culture, women have been portrayed too many times as emotional, hysterical, and at the mercy of the hormonal imbalances of our bodies. Several hundred years ago, women were buried alive or accused of witchcraft if they grew herbs or helped a sick neighbor. But healing and following life's natural cycles is part of our heritage as women of the earth. We give birth, we nurture and feed our young, we cool the fevered brow of a family member or friend, and we open our hearts to those around us. There are those who believe that the earth will not be able to heal until women reclaim their power as healers. Despite this awareness, we remain prey to a system of health care that does not honor our natural cycle of seasons. If we have too many complaints about ovarian or uterine pain, we are scheduled for a hysterectomy. If we don't deliver our babies fast enough, they give us a cesarean. If we go to the doctor too often, with too many complaints, we are given valium or Prozac. And by the time we make it to the autumn of our lives, we're given hormone replacement therapy that often makes us feel like there's something drastically wrong with the natural rhythm of menopause. In Asia, women rarely suffer from menopausal symptoms, breast cancer, PMS, or osteoporosis. Why? Some say it's the diet, some say it's cultural conditioning, and some say it's an honoring of the woman's natural progressions through life in the East.

"The biggest obstacle women face in healing/wellness is the belief that their bodies are defective or that they are victims of their body's symptoms," said Christiane Northrup, M.D., who cofounded Women to Women in Yarmouth, Maine and now spends much of her time educating women about the wisdom of their bodies. Dr. Northrup said women can begin the healing process by beginning to understand that their bodies contain a vast amount of inner wisdom, usually mediated through emotions, which are constantly broadcasting in which direction health lies in their lives. "Women can also begin to look at the wisdom encoded in their hormone fluctuations—monthly, during childbirth, and at menopause. In fact, it is my experience that those bodily processes we are taught to fear the most contain the most wisdom, and that includes the menstrual cycle, labor and delivery, breast feeding, and menopause."

Over the course of my reporting career I have interviewed countless women who have shared their feelings with me about their health care problems. It didn't even matter what their diagnosis was—MS, arthritis, carpal tunnel syndrome, headaches—they were often made to feel inferior to the doctor, made to feel as though all their physical symptoms were in their head, and as if they were helpless to improve their physical condition.

But many women are doing something about their health problems. They have researched alternatives on their own and found their own healing path. One woman shared that she had been telling doctors for months that she had cancer. They said she did not. Finally convinced that they were missing something, she got them to do elective surgery, and, sure enough, they had missed the cancer growing at the back of her tongue. This woman's internal healing instincts spoke to her; no one else heard her. Today she is teaching doctors in medical school how to listen to the patient and find the heart in healing.

"Healing is the filling-in of the hidden areas of a person's
life that are leading that person away from their full

*experience of health. So healing involves bringing these
areas into consciousness and transforming them. Often in
the process a physical cure takes place, but not always, and
therefore there needs to be a distinction between curing and
healing. We can often cure through surgery and drugs, which
simply means cutting out the affected part, or removing the
symptoms through pharmaceutical or even nutritional
means. Ultimately, however, this will not effect a complete
cure until the emotional, psychological, and spiritual aspects
of the condition are also addressed.*"

—Christiane Northrup, M.D.

CHILDBIRTH THE NATURAL WAY

*"When there are no complications or risks, I think that
a woman can do it all on her own, without any medical
interventions.*"

—Jacki Rooke, nurse midwife

Woman Discovers Her Birthing Path

After several hospital births, Mary was looking for an easier way. And
although she had never had any serious complications, she says she was
tired of the typical hospital interventions. Mary was tired of having her
labors induced by the pitocin drip just because she carried her babies
longer than the average 40 weeks.

"I just hated going to the hospital. I felt that I had no control. So in
my first trimester, I went to Jacki. At first she did not want to take me.
She said I was too high risk and that I wasn't in shape to give birth at
home. I changed my diet, eliminating processed foods and reducing
fat and sugar intake. And I started walking, gradually working up to
a mile every day. Two months later I went back to see Jacki and she
couldn't believe the change in me and my body. I felt much better and
I had a lot more energy," said Mary.

Now on her third home birth, Mary says the experiences have been
shockingly different, especially since her midwife has had children of her
own. Mary was quick to add that she's not a feminist, she is a traditional
conservative Christian, but being able to talk with a woman who under-
stands the birthing process is very different. Mary's husband also prefers

the home birth because in the hospital he felt restricted, and he was afraid to do anything. At home he is very comfortable working with his wife during her labor. One thing that could be a potential problem, Mary says, is that she has a tendency to give birth in the middle of major storms. So just to be safe, Jacki has an assistant on call who lives a mile away from Mary as the crow flies. It's Mary's pattern to go longer than the normal gestational time, but Jacki just lets her be, knowing this is her pattern. Mary sees home birth as by far the best alternative.

"Giving birth is something I look forward to. There are no pain-killers. It is a different kind of feeling, and at home I have more room to react to the pain. When you're lying flat, with tubes attached, you only have one way to react to your pain. It's very different when you have options."

Midwifery

Many women who have experienced home birth say that in a hospital they felt confined and forced to do things they didn't want to do. When the birthing process took too long, they were given a pitocin drip—that comes with its own set of problems like strengthening contractions before the baby is ready, and intensified pain—to speed up their labor. Many tell tales of cesarean sections that they believe were not necessary.

> "A fundamental alteration in the attitude of physician and patient toward the management of childbirth has come about during the present generation. It is a surgical procedure and as such can best be dealt with in a hospital."
>
> —Barton Cooke Hirst, 1925, the founder of one of the first maternity hospitals in the country

When doctors and hospitals started to encourage women to give birth in the hospital instead of home, some women protested, and home births were still prominent in this country well into the early part of this century. This transition—from home to hospital—had considerable social implications. It virtually collapsed ancient customs and centuries-old traditions of women and midwives helping each other during the birthing process. Now men were in charge, controlling this natural process, and the protests of women were discounted. It wasn't until the past few years that midwives could legally operate in many states.

Jacki Rooke is a certified nurse midwife, and although she runs her own birthing center in Charlottesville, Virginia, she still delivers some babies at home for women who request a home birth. Jacki's been helping women give birth for most of her nursing career. She believes that childbirth is an experience that must happen in a supportive environment. And try as the doctors and staff might, there are just too many rules in hospitals for deliveries to work in the natural way.

Jacki says it's been a hard road. "When I started thirteen years ago, I couldn't find a doctor to back me up," she says. Now under the supervision of an obstetrician, Jacki always has backup medical support in case of emergencies. She prepares her women for birth as if they were in training for a marathon, encouraging daily exercise and improved diets, because she believes that women must be in shape. She says that if women are prepared and in a comfortable, stress-free environment, their labor is much easier.

Jacki's birthing center is in a red brick home in a suburban neighborhood, just north of the Blue Ridge Mountains. It's warm and inviting, and it could be anybody's home. Only the more than double-sized Jacuzzi near the bed gives any clue that this might not be the guest bedroom. I must admit, I was wishing I had been able to deliver my own children this way. Jacki says women love the tub, and she chose a big one in order to give them space to move with their contractions. "The hospital's Jacuzzis are so small, the women, especially pregnant women, can't move in them." Many times the woman's partner will get in the tub with her to help her through the labor. Jacki says the woman can do what she wants in her time, and that in itself makes the birth more natural, more like what ancient wisdom taught us.

Some Tips for a Better Birthing Experience

- An acupuncturist can alleviate the pain of labor and can often help women who have a history of difficult labors. If this is something you desire, you will have to talk to an acupuncturist early in your pregnancy and then obtain the necessary permission for a home birth from either a midwife or the hospital.
- If you are prone to nausea, have an acupuncturist show you the acupressure point on your wrist that relieves nausea. It's on the underside of the forearm, about 1 1/2 inches from your wrist. Just press it with your thumb for about ten to fifteen counts and release. Repeat several times.
- Make certain you feel comfortable with the environment you will give birth in.

- During pregnancy, exercise three times a week. Walking is wonderful exercise.
- Watch your intake of sugars, fats, and salt and try to keep them low.
- Ask your health care practitioner about taking PN-6 capsules when you are close to your due date. This herbal combination softens and thins the cervix, which helps the cervix dilate and often shortens labor.
- Drink raspberry tea or pregnancy tea in the last two months to tonify the uterus. Some say it shortens labor.
- Make sure you only invite people to your delivery who you want to be there. This is *your* birth experience.
- If you've had other children, sit down and write what you felt like during the various stages of labor. What did you like? What did you hate? In what way do you want your partner to participate? And then make sure someone can see that your wishes are carried out.
- Alfalfa and zinc help keep your energy level up, but check with your health care practitioner first.
- Extract of gotu kola can help heal an episiotomy.

Herbs for Pregnancy

Because each pregnancy is very different, it is best to talk to your health care provider before taking any of these herbs while pregnant.

MORNING SICKNESS

A cup of ginger root tea or a few ginger capsules can help. Also peppermint tea and a short nap helps. My daughter suffered miserably from nausea in the beginning of her second pregnancy. I would give her a cup of peppermint tea and have her take a short nap. She always woke up feeling better. You can also chew on anise seeds.

LABOR

During the eighth month, begin drinking several cups of raspberry tea per day. In ancient times, once in labor women used herbs such as blue cohosh and raspberry leaves to bring on stronger uterine contractions. Rosemary, lavender, and chamomile essential oil rubbed on the wrists and other pulse points eases labor pains.

BREAST FEEDING

Dill and anise increase milk production. Two teaspoons of dill or one teaspoon of anise made into a tea and taken three times a day will help considerably. Some also suggest nettle to aid in breast feeding.

PMS: BLOATED, CRABBY, AND CRAVING

Most of us have been there, like addicts looking for a fix, we're tearing up the cupboards searching for that piece of chocolate we hid the last time the cravings started. And when it's really bad, it's not just the chocolate, it's the salty chips, too. I had a friend who would just salt the chocolate, and that tastes about the same! There were times that the cravings and the water weight gain just about drove me crazy. It's hormones, they would tell me. But I wanted to do something to stop it. It just didn't seem normal. Then about ten years ago a nurse practitioner told me about vitamin B-complex. I take one every day, and I move in and out of my menstrual cycles with ease. The Chinese say that diet dramatically effects hormones, and a diet high in animal-based foods will elevate hormones, which increases the likelihood that you will have problems with PMS and menopause. According to researchers for the China Project (see Chapter Seven), diets rich in dark green vegetables, whole grains, and legumes provide magnesium and vitamin B6, which are said to reduce PMS symptoms. In Chinese medicine, women experiencing premenstrual symptoms or painful periods have been treated successfully more than 85 percent of the time with acupuncture and Chinese herbs.

Food and PMS

The following foods can help reduce or alleviate the symptoms of PMS:

> Foods containing calcium are said to reduce mood swings. Yogurt is good.
>
> Complex carbohydrates (especially whole grains), studies show, alleviate the symptoms of PMS.
>
> Soybeans and soy products.
>
> Seek out foods high in manganese, such as pineapple, vegetables, grains, nuts, seeds, and tea.

Herbs and PMS

Evening Primrose: Studies in England have shown that women with severe PMS have been helped by taking three capsules a day of evening primrose oil starting the three days prior to the normal onset of PMS and continuing until menstruation.

False Unicorn: Treats cramps.

Valerian: This herb has an overall calming effect and eases cramps.

Dong quai: Treats cramps.

White willow: Alleviates headache and cramps.

Chamomile tea: Chamomile tea is a general soother.

Prozac the Natural Way

St. John's Wort, an herb that's been around for centuries, is said to relieve mild to moderate depression as well as the popular pharmaceutical preparations like Prozac. According to the *British Medical Journal,* researchers studied ten years' worth of research on St. John's Wort, and the results of the majority of the fifteen studies that compared the evergreen plant to a placebo indicated that it was as effective as the anti-depressants currently being prescribed. In Germany in 1993 more than 3 million prescriptions were written for St. John's Wort for individuals suffering from mild depression, sleep problems, and anxiety. In 1997 the National Institutes of Health, Office of Alternative Medicine and the Office of Dietary Supplements began collaborating to fund research on the benefits of the herb.

MENOPAUSE

Menopause is part of the natural progression of a woman's life, generally beginning its gradual course when a woman reaches her late forties or early fifties, although the age of onset varies. It is a time when a woman passes from the reproductive to nonreproductive years of her life. In the years or months leading up to menopause, the ovaries' production of estrogen slows, often causing hormones to fluctuate. Menstrual periods become irregular, and some women may also experience insomnia, hot flashes, night sweats, depression, frequent urination or urinary incontinence, vaginal dryness, and a change in sexual desire. These symptoms, more typical in American women, rarely affect Asian women, who have few problems with passage into this phase of life.

Menopause does not have to be difficult. In Eastern cultures it is viewed as a very natural progression in a woman's life and seasonal cycles. If problems with menopause do arise in Asian women, the t riggering factor is often viewed as an imbalance between the liver and kidneys, with a weakness in the kidneys and a deficiency in the blood. Acupuncture needling is often very effective in reestablishing the balance. And occasionally herbal treatment is also used to restore hormonal balance, including Chinese angelica root, peony root, thorowax root, and raw or cooked rehmannia.

The China Project (see Chapter Seven) also reported that plant foods, especially soy products, contain plant estrogens that provide a natural source of estrogen, an important dietary consideration since a woman's estrogen levels fall naturally during menopause. Some researchers believe that a high intake of soy—tofu, miso, and soybean juice—may explain why an Asian woman's passage into midlife is often symptom-free.

Herbs and Menopause

Chinese Angelica root (*Angelica sinensis*) is a female tonic and helps alleviate vaginal dryness.

Ginseng tea can relieve hot flashes and other symptoms.

There are also preparations of such things as valerian, dong quai, black cohosh, and licorice that can help menopausal symptoms.

Other options for treating the symptoms of menopause:

- Oil of evening primose
- Magnesium
- Zinc
- Iron
- Vitamin B6, vitamin B-Complex, and vitamins C and E
- Lemongrass baths
- Diets low in caffeine and high in soy and tofu
- Jojoba oil to counter vaginal dryness prior to intercourse
- Rose oil or diluted tea tree oil baths
- Meditation, exercise, and yoga

Current Studies on the Use of Herbs to Treat Menopausal Symptoms

The College of Physicians and Surgeons at Columbia-Presbyterian Medical Center in collaboration with Georgetown University Medical

Center and the Taoist Health Institute are currently conducting a clinical trial to study the effectiveness of an herbal formula for reducing the frequency and severity of menopausal hot flashes. Although Columbia researchers would not reveal the names of the herbs in the combination, they did say that this formula has been used in China for centuries. This clinical trial, which has not yet been completed, is funded by a pilot grant from the National Institutes of Health, Office of Alternative Medicine, and the principal investigator is Fredi Kronenberg, Ph.D., the director of the Richard and Hinda Rosenthal Center for Alternative/Complementary Medicine at Columbia. The Columbia study is the first double-blind, placebo-controlled, crossover clinical trial to assess the effect of Chinese herbs on hot flashes. The herbs were formulated at East Earth Herb Inc., in Eugene, Oregon and, according to researchers, the formula to be studied was described in 1253 and modified in 1509 by Sue Ji in "Annotations on Good Prescriptions for Women." Dr. Kronenberg says, "Many women experiment on their own with vitamin E, or various herbal preparations that they hear about by word of mouth. These preparations have not been studied in a systematic way for their effect on hot flashes or for possible adverse effects. It is important to explore natural medicinals used in other cultures, since we may find new ways to help those women for whom hot flashes are so disabling."

DONG QUAI: A POSSIBLE ALTERNATIVE TO ESTROGEN

A first-time clinical study sponsored by Kaiser Permanente on the benefits of *dong quai* for menopausal women may offer hope to women not wanting hormone replacement therapy. Dong quai, a Chinese herb, has been used in that country for centuries by Asian women as a tonic to relieve menstrual irregularities and to treat menopausal symptoms such as mood swings, loss of vitality, hot flashes, and insomnia.

As with soy foods, which are also beneficial for menopausal symptoms, dong quai is rich in natural chemicals that resemble estrogens. According to the study's lead researcher, Bruce Ettinger, M.D., president of the North American Menopause Society, the purpose of the study is not to find a replacement for estrogen, but rather to verify the centuries-old anecdotal evidence of the efficacy of dong quai.

> "The interest in dong quai reflects profound changes in so-
> cial and medical attitudes toward menopause. It's a natural
> process in a woman's life."
>
> —Bruce Ettinger, M.D.

Osteoporosis and Calcium

Admittedly, I was surprised when reviewing the results of the China Project (Chapter Seven) to discover that a connection was made between low dairy intake and low levels of osteoporosis. In fact, according to the study, the incidence of hip fractures in China is one-fifth of that in the West. Coming from a long line of osteoporosis sufferers, this was very interesting information. For years we've been told, "Eat more dairy and get more calcium." What I wasn't told was that certain foods, like animal protein, can actually deplete calcium from our bones, and a high protein diet can cause the body to excrete more calcium than it actually takes in. This is important information for a country in which nearly 25 million people suffer from this degenerative bone-thinning disease.

Foods that contain the trace element boron can help the body hold on to calcium and prevent this debilitating condition. According to researchers at the U.S. Department of Agriculture's Human Nutrition Research Center in North Dakota, a deficiency in boron can hamper calcium metabolism, causing brittle bones. Some boron-rich foods are fruit, nuts, apples, pears, grapes, dates, raisins, peaches, legumes, soybeans, and honey. Also the herb horsetail helps the body absorb calcium.

If you are seeking calcium-enhancing foods other than dairy products, try: broccoli, tofu, soybeans, pinto beans, chickpeas, okra, kale, dried figs, raisins, dates, white beans, pineapple, and pineapple juice.

WOMEN NEED TO THINK TWICE ABOUT UNNECESSARY AND HARMFUL TREATMENTS

- More than 20 million American women have had a hysterectomy, and 600,000 procedures are added to the toll each year.
- More than 500,000 unnecessary cesarean births are performed each year in this country. The U.S. cesarean birth rate is nearly three times that of Japan.
- Women get twice as many prescriptions for tranquilizers and sleeping pills—about 66 million—than men do.

TEN

Healing through Energy, Touch, and Gentle Exercise

*"My parents are both deceased, I had lost a child, and
I felt kind of alone in the world. Like everything was
on my shoulders. Karen helped me with that load. She
would touch me and her touching said, yes, I care. And
that's what healing is all about."*

—Cindy, 37, Pennsylvania

For centuries, touch has been an important part of healing. The hands
were the physician's eyes, diagnosing and treating. But now, in this technologically advanced era of medicine, a physician rarely touches the
patient. We're covered with lead aprons, and the technician stands
behind a shield. The chasm between healer and patient grows increasingly larger with threats of malpractice suits looming and doctors being
squeezed by the capitation rates set by bean counters at the insurance
companies.

LIFE FORCE AROUND THE GLOBE

Most cultures have a name for the body's energy. Here is a list of some
of the names used by cultures old and new:

Ancient Egypt, Ankh; Ancient Greece, Pneuma; China, qi; Dakota,
Ton; Ghana, Mulungu; Hawaii, Tane; Huron, Oki; India, Prana; Iro-
quois, Orenda; Japan, Ki; Lakota, Wakan; Mesmer, Animal magnet-
ism; United States and United Kingdom, Bioenergy, Subtle Energy,
and Biomagnetism.

Biofield Healing

Energy healing or the laying on of hands, also called *biofield therapeutics,* is one of the oldest forms of healing, dating back to the mythical Yellow Emperor in China and hieroglyphic recordings from Egypt's Third Dynasty. Hippocrates referred to the force from the healer's hands, giving this therapeutic connection a great deal of attention.

There are two schools of thought about energy healing: some believe that the healing force comes from a source other than the practitioner, such as the universe or God (see Chapter Eleven); others attribute the source to the human biofield, an energy source or field that encircles and permeates living bodies, also known as qi or the life force. Therapeutic application of the biofield is when the practitioner places his or her hands on or near the patient. Some practitioners work on the assumption that the field extends beyond the body for several inches, so they believe that holding their hands above the body is as effective as actually touching the patient. And it is in the union of the two energies that healing occurs. Taking a holistic approach, generally energy practitioners treat the mental, spiritual, and physical body. Several studies have been conducted on biofield treatment, including measuring the voltage readings (see Chapter Five) from the healer's hands during the treatment. In recent years, many Western-trained nurses have become practiced in therapeutic touch to heal their patients in ways that medicine or surgery cannot. Some of the biofield therapies used in the United States include qigong (Chinese), Reiki (Japanese), therapeutic touch (United States), healing touch (American Holistic Nurses Association), Huna (Hawaiian), healing science (United States).

> "The ability to heal is a natural human potential. Healing itself is the conscious, full engagement of the therapist's own access to vital energy flows in the compassionate interest of helping another who is ill. Healing, then, can be thought of as a humanization of energy."
>
> —Dolores Krieger, Ph.D., R.N.,
> author of *Accepting Your Power to Heal:*
> *The Personal Practice of Therapeutic Touch*

CLINICAL PROMISE FOR ENERGY HEALING

Out of eighteen clinical studies conducted on humans, 56 percent of individuals participating in the research showed significant results and improved health status after treatments involving energy healing. Some areas in which research has demonstrated clinical and therapeutic promise are in reducing anxiety, reducing acute and chronic pain, speeding up the healing of wounds, healing after surgery, speeding up healing for thermal burns and decreasing pain, treating migraines, alleviating PMS, treating panic attacks, treating post-traumatic stress disorder, treating irritable bowel syndrome, easing the third trimester of pregnancy and the birthing process, treating eating disorders, fighting addictions, treating sexual dysfunction.

REIKI: THE LAYING ON OF HANDS

As ancient lore tells the tale, *reiki* (pronounced *ray-key*), a Japanese word meaning "universal life," evolved from Tibetan Buddhism. Its healing properties are based on the invisible flow of energy in all living things. Passed from master to disciple, reiki involves the passing of energy from the healer to the healee, and it is generally intended to promote physical, emotional, and spiritual peace. For several centuries, the ancient secrets of this Tibetan practice were lost. It wasn't until the nineteenth century that Dr. Mikao Usui, a Japanese Buddhist monk, on a spiritually healing quest, revived the lost art. According to historical writings, Dr. Usai spent fourteen years on this sacred journey. It is said that following a three-week mountaintop meditation, Dr. Usai had a vision of four healing symbols, which formed the basis for the reiki legacy. And reiki healers were able to channel their energy to others only after finding attunement to the four symbols. Before his death, Dr. Usai trained sixteen masters in the reiki secrets of attunement.

Reiki is still practiced in Japan but wasn't introduced in America until 1936, when the first reiki clinic was opened in Hawaii. Today there are more than 200,000 reiki practitioners. There are different spiritual levels of specialty in the reiki passage to master level, and before going to a reiki healer you may choose to inquire about that practitioner's lineage, so that you have an idea of the strength of the tradition he or she has been schooled in. According to preliminary data, emotional, physical, and spiritual conditions respond well to reiki, but the extent of the healing depends on the connection between the healer and the healee, including the patient's willingness to participate in his or her own healing journey.

The treatment process will vary somewhat from one healer to the next, but generally you get on the treatment table, often a massage table, fully clothed, and you lie down. After covering you with a soft sheet, the reiki practitioner begins the treatment, often to music. Sitting at the head of the table, the healer touches the head *chakra* (chakras were first defined in ancient Indian practices; they are areas of rotation in the biofield). The healer's touch is gentle, and you barely notice it, other than having an occasional warm feeling. Moving down the body to cover all the chakras, the reiki healer is silent during this loving exchange. It takes about half an hour, and following the session the reiki practitioner will share any insights that may have been revealed during the exchange. Physical reactions to reiki treatment are very different, depending on the person: some people fall asleep, some have vivid images of known or unknown events, and others describe soothing feelings or images of color or nature.

Reiki Treatment for a Mother-to-Be

Thirty-seven-year-old Cindy turned to reiki to heal a painful loss. A loss she blames on herself. Two years earlier, she had been pregnant with her second child. But at twenty-six weeks, her blood pressure shot up and just stayed there. Finally admitting her to the hospital for preeclampsia (a serious condition that is more common in women with diabetes, high blood pressure, or kidney disease), Cindy's doctor recommended all the conventional precautions: bed rest, regular monitoring. "The nurses kept telling me everything was alright," she recalls, the pain still evident in her voice. "But I knew something was wrong, and three days later there was no heartbeat." Collin died.

Cindy and her husband live in a medium-size southeastern Pennsylvania industrial city. Like many living in what could be defined as blue-collar America, the couple operates a family-owned business, and much of their life is taken up by work, family, and simple pleasures. Perhaps to make up for the death of Collin, she and her husband hoped she would become pregnant again. But in light of her past medical history and the trouble she was having trying to conceive following Collin's death, doctors advised that she and her husband adopt.

For Cindy, this wasn't the answer. Seeking the advice of specialists, Cindy talked to and was examined by some of the best. Despite their intervention and her desire to bring another life into the world, her womb remained empty. On the suggestion of her internist, who was helping keep her blood pressure under control, Cindy went to a counselor who in turn suggested that Cindy try reiki therapy. Cindy admits that she had never heard of such a thing and was skeptical. She made an appointment to visit Karen Sweitzer, a reiki master who has studied with Deepak Chopra and Steven Covey. When she arrived for her appointment, Cindy says she kept looking around the room and thinking, "What am I doing? Why am I here?" But because of her condition, she had a high stake in the therapy being a success, even though she kept thinking she must be crazy.

The reiki room, located in a back corner of Karen Sweitzer's middle-class, suburban brick-frame home, is filled with the wonderful scents of spice, earth, and love. Karen's voice is soothing—soft, kind. And she always starts her sessions with shared conversation and a cup of warmed water. For Cindy, Karen turned out to be the right prescription.

When Cindy got up on the reiki table, Karen covered her with a soft flannel sheet. Sitting at her head, Karen began. Cindy says that her first experience was profound, but she did not share this with Karen. Cindy was still feeling guarded, and, besides, she hoped Karen would not see the emotion swelling inside her. She wrote about her reiki experience in her journal as soon as she returned home:

"When she touched my head I saw a tunnel. I didn't plan for this. It was so emotional. It was a dark tunnel, and I could see lights. I thought about my baby, and I knew he was with me. I saw a blazing light and fireworks. I felt such extreme emotions, and I hoped she didn't see me. I could feel my womb tensing, and I knew that this was the place that my baby had died."

Cindy decided to continue seeing Karen for reiki sessions. At the same time, she discovered that she was pregnant—something Karen had sensed during the first reiki treatment. With the help of a new obstetrician and weekly visits to Karen, Cindy's blood pressure remained normal throughout her pregnancy.

Karen reached out to Cindy, offering her positive healing energy. She even stayed by Cindy's side at ultrasound exams and during her labor. Cindy says it was very important that the baby be born naturally, and Karen encouraged her to talk to her baby. Cindy did. Nolan came quickly, two hours after labor began: no medication, no complications. Cindy credits Karen with helping her release old pains, leaving her free to love again.

*"I felt that she had breathed life into me. I felt strong again.
I was calmer, more relaxed, and every time I left [after a
reiki session] I felt right with the world. She helped me talk
to my baby, and I could tell in her voice that she cared
about me and was telling me about myself."*

—Cindy, 37, Pennsylvania

BALANCING THE CHI THROUGH GENTLE EXERCISES

T'ai-Chi Ch'uan

They move with grace, ease and precision. Feeling the connection to the universe; the air, the earth, their breath, they dance in ease to the cycles of nature in this moving meditation. More Americans are learning the ancient martial art form of T'ai-Chi Ch'uan (tye jee). In China or California, city parks are lined with people rooted in the silent strength of gentle, flowing motion.

T'ai-Chi Ch'uan was founded by Chang San-feng in the fourteenth century. It consists of a set of graceful movements, like a slow dance. It has been called shadow boxing. The movements encourage the free flow of chi through the meridians, improving circulation. The concentration and relaxed but mindful breathing help bring on a state of relaxation and a more positive mood.

T'ai-Chi has its origin in Taoism, an integral part of Chinese philosophy. The word tao means "road" or "path," and t'ai-chi reflects a path to wisdom through listening, observing, and feeling. According to Tricia Yu, a T'ai-Chi instructor in Madison, Wisconsin, who learned the art of T'ai-Chi twenty-three years ago, "Legend has it that T'ai-Chi emerged around the twelfth century, A.D. in Taoist hermitages. Taoists see man as a microcosm of the universe and the body as a reflection of one's attunement of the cycles, rhythms, and patterns of the larger universe. The people who created T'ai-Chi lived simple, secluded lives, gardening and gathering food from the wild. They observed the cycles of nature on earth, while watching and recording the patterns and pathways of the stars. They spent hours meditating, feeling and observing their own bodies, noting the rhythms, currents, and connections within. For exercise, they practiced the martial arts—man-to-man combat—and watched all living creatures, how they moved, how they reacted to danger, and how they defended themselves. Perhaps because of the quiet simplicity of their lives and their single-minded intent to probe beyond the immediately apparent, these people attained a high degree of body awareness, intuitive attunement, and a valuable body knowledge about nature and her cycles, and a cosmology that is compatible with modern theoretical physics."

THE YANG STYLE

According to Lee Felton, a body worker and T'ai-Chi instructor with Blue Ridge Chi, in Charlottesville, Virginia, a branch of the New York

School of T'ai-Chi Ch'uan, the various styles of T'ai-Chi evolved over generations through different families. As legend goes, these families were mandated to teach the nobility what had been in their family for many years. That is how the public and secret forms of T'ai-Chi came about. The public version was more diluted, he says. Over time the traditional Yang family form of T'ai-Chi was modified and is known today as the Yang Style, short form; it basically got rid of repetition. T'ai-Chi today is a shadow of what it once was, according to Felton, although masters retain some of their self in the style they teach.

STUDIES ON THE EFFICACY OF T'AI-CHI

Three Virginia Beach physical therapists conducted a study on the effect of yang style T'ai-Chi on balance-impaired individuals. And according to their study, this Chinese martial art has positive implications in the practice of physical therapy. All subjects underwent an initial pretest of balance ability, followed by semi-weekly sessions of T'ai-Chi (Yang form) led by Lawrence Mann, a T'ai-Chi instructor who is now deceased, for six weeks. During that time the subjects completed seven of the sixty or seventy T'ai-Chi postures. At the twelfth session, the subjects' balance was reevaluated.[1]

The results were significant on the postural sway—the way the body moves—with eyes closed, says Rebecca Phalen, MPT. "But we needed more time. The subjects still needed verbal instruction and had not yet incorporated T'ai-Chi into their daily routine." Nonetheless, according to Phalen, the anecdotal evidence was incredible. Subjects and families reported that they felt more confident, and more than 50 percent of the participants decided to continue their study of t'ai chi. "This practice has been around for centuries, and I think that it is something that we can incorporate into our treatments. Both bodies of knowledge, when used together, can better benefit the patient," says Phalen.

According to Tricia Yu, T'ai-Chi Ch'uan is a weight-bearing and moderate-intensity cardiovascular exercise that can improve balance, reduce falls, and increase leg strength as well as lower stress hormones, enhance respiratory and immune function, and promote emotional well-being. Recently several studies have examined the implications of older people (age seventy and older) practicing T'ai-Chi. The results of these studies indicate that this gentle Chinese exercise has a positive effect on biomedical and psychosocial indices of frailty; favorably affects the occurrence of falls; increases strength; may delay the decline of cardiorespiratory function; may be prescribed as a suitable aerobic exercise for older adults; improves functional balance and postural control.

The ROM Dance

First developed in 1981, by Tricia Yu, M.A., health educator and Diane Harlowe, M.S., occupational therapist, the ROM (Range Of Motion) Dance is now recommended by doctors and therapists for people with pain and physical limitations. The ROM Dance combines Western medical model range of motion exercises with Eastern-based T'ai-Chi, qigong, and meditative poems. It gained increased credibility following the National Arthritis Foundation stamp of approval. Historically, the rote range of motion exercises usually prescribed by physical and occupational therapists can be boring and painful for patients. That's why Yu and Harlowe decided to combine their Eastern and Western knowledge to make the necessary exercises better for their patients, and to improve the chances that patients would keep up with their exercises once they went home from the hospitals. From the very first studies conducted by the Arthritis Foundation, patient compliance improved considerably. Participants say they would much rather catch a sunbeam than concentrate on shoulder flexion.

"I am sitting on my chair at a quiet beach. The sun is shining brightly. Warm waves lap at my feet as they dangle in the water. . . . I scoop the water over my head, covering me with a warm waterfall. . ." and so begins the series of movements that seem graceful and inviting and peaceful. The ROM Dance is the first holistic approach to range of motion exercises.

Based on movements first developed for rheumatoid arthritis, the ROM Dance has been expanded and is now being used to help patients with fibromyalgia; hand problems; cancer; Parkinson's disease; neurological problems; pain management; stress management; and psychiatric and geriatric issues. Yu says that the ROM Dance meditative poem was changed for use with lupus patients. The original meditative poem talks of bathing in warm sunlight, something that is deadly to people with lupus, so the dance was altered to ROM Dance by Moonlight. The first poem, which was added near the end of the dance's creation, appealed to women more than men, says Yu. Wanting to reach both audiences, she and Harlowe also have a version that has a meditative journey by the campfire for men.

Yu composed the piano music for the dance, and she and Harlowe co-created the poem and movements, which are available on video and audiotape. In therapy pockets around the country, therapists are now trained in the ROM Dance technique, and according to Yu, the ROM Dance Network was formed to help meet the increasing need for training from these two educators in Madison, Wisconsin.

THE SEVEN PRINCIPLES OF THE ROM DANCE

- attention to the present
- diaphragmatic deep breathing
- postural alignment
- relaxed movement
- slow movement
- awareness of movement
- imagination

Qigong

Qigong, (*chee-gung*), known in China as longevity and health exercises, combines graceful, physical movements with mental concentration. In the practice of qigong, the gentle movements, while appearing similar to those in T'ai-Chi, do not flow from one to the other as in T'ai-Chi. Rather, they are done in shorter movement groups and are repeated many times. With T'ai-Chi it can take anywhere from several months to over a year to grasp the rudimentary principles; qigong can be learned more quickly. And like T'ai-Chi, quigong can be modified, so that even very ill individuals can do the exercises. In recent years, this very gentle exercise has been used to help AIDS patients. George Wedemeyer and Emelio Gonzalez, both HIV-positive, credit their longevity to the daily practice of qigong (see Chapter Five). Several years ago, the two developed a gentler approach to the qigong movements.

According to Traditional Chinese Medicine, health is restored when the body's qi is flowing and balanced. Qigong gentle exercises are actually slow, fluid movements that reduce stress and are designed to balance the body's energy along the meridians.

In recent years, the Chinese have been studying the long-term effects of qigong on medical conditions, in particular, cancer, AIDS, and arthritis, as well as its effect on the body's nervous, respiratory, circulatory, digestive, endocrine, and immune systems. Although the studies are preliminary, it has been determined that qigong can lower heart rates, slow breathing, control blood pressure, induce a deeper state of relaxation, improve cardiopulmonary circulation, produce a massaging effect on the intestines and help the digestive process, lower glucose levels in diabetics, and noticeably affect the immune system.[2]

ELEVEN

Shooting Up: Treating Substance Abuse with Acupuncture and Community Solutions

"I believe you are addicted long before you pick up your first drug. And you can be clean and miserable. Acupuncture teaches you how to heal from the inside out."

—Hebrew Watson, former heroin addict

Addiction is familiar to all of us. Either we have had a problem with a substance or an activity or we know someone who has been affected by such a problem. Given that more than one in four Americans is dependent on something—illegal drugs, prescription drugs, alcohol, food, sex, gambling, the Internet, tobacco, caffeine—it's fairly likely that someone in your family, a friend, a neighbor, or a co-worker is addicted. The cost in lives, chronic health conditions, crime, lost work time, and broken families is staggering. Addictions afflict the poor and the well off, people of all ages and all kinds of circumstances.

General Motors estimates that it is spending over $1 billion a year on substance abuse-related expenses for its employees. In Flint, Michigan, the automaker began using the acupuncture treatment model on an outpatient basis to treat employee addiction. General Motors tracked the results of the treatment and found that 83 percent of a group of one hundred employees were clean, productive, and reliable workers one year after entering acupuncture treatment.

THE EXPERIENCE OF A HEALING HEROIN ADDICT

Hebrew Watson says there is a better way. And he should know, he has been using heroin on and off for twenty-five years. He says that last year he found something that has helped him face his disease head-on for the first time—acupuncture.

The forty-three-year-old recovering addict discovered this alternative to conventional addiction treatment at Baltimore's Penn North Neighborhood Center, which, with the assistance of the Traditional Acupuncture Institute in Columbia, Maryland, offers a program that incorporates Chinese medicine for the treatment of addictions. Patients like Hebrew are finding hope and healing through the Center's treatment plan, which combines Twelve-step programs, acupuncture and herbs, counseling, and nutrition with strategies for reintegrating addicts into their community.

According to Hebrew, many of the detox programs that he'd been through in the past helped him get off the drugs, but there didn't seem to be anything to help him with the problems that come with withdrawal, such as not being able to sleep; having drug dreams; suffering from body aches; foggy head, and tension headaches; and not being able to focus. Hebrew reports that acupuncture helped alleviate these problems, so he could concentrate on what he was being taught about his body and his addiction. In the past, when he tried to get clean, all these physical problems got in the way of him staying off heroin.

ACUPUNCTURE AND ADDICTION

Jody Forman, a licensed acupuncturist who previously worked for the National Institute on Drug Abuse and the U.S. Department of Justice and has worked in the field of addictions for the better part of her career, sees acupuncture as an excellent complement to conventional treatment for addiction. Not only does it help patients respond better to counseling and lifestyle changes; it is a very economical means of treating large numbers of patients.

Addictions treatment is a very difficult proposition, those seeking treatment often have a lot of regrets, and they have a very strong pull to

One of the big things in treatment is to get the patients to stay in treatment.

get high again. Acupuncture essentially does what the drug does for them. It calms and quiets their mind, which helps to keep them in treatment long enough to learn.

Methadone is still used to treat heroin addiction, but unfortunately, once patients get on methadone, they rarely ever get off it. Practitioners of alternative treatments for addicts consider the use of methadone the substitution of one addiction with another. According to a 1995 report from the Alcohol and Drug Abuse Administration, individuals on methadone treatment spend more time in treatment and leave treatment drug-free less frequently than do patients involved in any other form of addiction treatment program. According to the report, the average duration of methadone treatment in the state of Maryland is 3.7 years. And the cost of methadone treatment is approximately $3,286 per year as compared to about $250 to $1,000 for acupuncture treatment.

Most alternative addiction treatment programs follow the treatment protocol of the National Acupuncture Detoxification Association (NADA), which formed in 1985. (*Alternative* is actually a misnomer, since this type of treatment is so widely used today.) Merging the field's of acupuncture and addictions treatment, NADA established standards to assure the best possible care and treatment for patients in this new modality. The standard treatment protocol involves ear acupuncture needling consisting of five acupuncture points on the ear.

In Chinese theory, the practitioner treating addiction works to build the yin energy. The yin energy is the cooling, quiet energy that can restore the patient to better health. Yang energy is more like the energy of the hyper, Type-A personality, according to Jody Forman. When lifestyle or substances deplete or burn up the yin, it needs to be restored to rebalance the yin and yang. A yin deficiency is often referred to as empty fire. According to Dr. Michael Smith of the Lincoln Hospital drug treatment program in the South Bronx (discussed later in this chapter), many addicts have false fire attitudes, illusions of power that lead them to engage in more desperate drug abuse and senseless violence. Acupuncture is an effective means of treating empty fire conditions. By restoring or tonifying yin, the patient is empowered in a soft, gentle manner.

Balls and Seeds

Some acupuncturists use small metal balls or seeds taped to acupuncture points on the patient's ear to help the addict when he or she is not at the treatment center. Forman says she prefers to use vaccarria seeds, derived from the black radish plant, for this purpose. This method is very effective for those trying to quit smoking, according to Forman. Following acupuncture needling, the seeds are attached to the acupuncture points in the ear with surgical tape. When the patient has a craving, he or she rubs and presses on the seeds to stop the craving.

The Lincoln Hospital Program Was the Forerunner

Setting the path for others, under the direction of Michael Smith, M.D., certified acupuncturist, the Lincoln Hospital in the South Bronx, previously known as a methadone and detoxification clinic for this ghetto neighborhood, started administering acupuncture to hard-core addicts in 1974. About five years later, methadone was no longer on the clinic's protocol for treatment of heroin addicts. According to Dr. Smith, hard-core addicts are generally shocked to discover that daily acupuncture can relieve withdrawal as reliably as the drugs they were using.

Since more than 200 patients were seeking treatment each day, Dr. Smith was able to gather a great deal of data about the effectiveness of this type of treatment, which he says provides an excellent guiding principal in helping people participate in their own recovery.

Dr. Smith says acupuncture alleviates some of the chronic tension, cravings, and insomnia that accompany withdrawal from the toxic substance. These symptoms, according to Eastern theory, reflect an imbalance in the body's qi. Once the qi gets back in balance, patients often say they no longer have a desire to drink or use drugs, and the painful symptoms associated with getting off the drugs disappear. As a result patients are better able to concentrate, so they can learn about their addiction, their body and how to make changes in their life. Dr. Smith says that it is important to integrate acupuncture treatment with counseling (with trained addictions counselors) to balance the body, the mind, and psychosocial issues. Patients come to Lincoln to be treated for abusing alcohol, heroin, cocaine, methadone, sedatives, stimulants, and hallucinogens.

The principals and protocols set forth at Lincoln Hospital have served as the foundation for more than eight hundred other clinics around the world, including Hungary, London, Saudi Arabia, Trinidad, and Katmandu, according to Dr. Smith. Programs following close on the heels of Lincoln were established in Brooklyn and Minneapolis. The Brooklyn program, established in 1983 as part of Kings County Hospital Substance Abuse Services, demonstrated impressive results.

Studies on the Efficacy of Acupuncture in Treating Substance Abuse

LINCOLN HOSPITAL STUDIES

In a summary of treatment studies, Dr. Smith reported the following findings in testimony before the U.S. Congress.

- Ninety percent relief of symptoms in acute withdrawal clients.
- Ninety percent of those who come for acupuncture treatment return for further treatment without any other incentives or pressures.
- Sixty percent of those treated remained drug-free six months after completing the program.
- Among clients on probation from the criminal justice system, those treated with acupuncture were discharged early from their probation five times more often than those who were not treated with acupuncture.
- According to Dr. Smith, "Without exception, the clients interviewed were enthusiastic about acupuncture. Many remarked they were less tense, less fearful and able to cope with things a lot better."[1]

OTHER STUDIES

In a study of 90 Kings County alcoholism clients who were referred for acupuncture treatment because of regular positive Breathalyzer tests, 60 of these patients had ongoing negative Breathalyzer tests since their first day of treatment with acupuncture. According to data in the study, these patients had not been functioning members of society, but, following treatment, many went on to become leading models of sobriety, often counseling others.

The Department of Toxicology at Hennepin County Medical Center in Minneapolis conducted a controlled evaluation of acupuncture treatment for chronic abusers. In the study, placebo acupuncture points, which were 1–3 millimeters away from the actual point, were used for one group. The others received acupuncture needling at the five correct points in the ear. Researchers chose the patients based on frequent inpatient detoxification failures. These patients all lived in the same facility and received no other treatment. Patients were told they could drink and were given free bus tokens, so they had access to area bars. According to the findings, there was a significant difference between the actual and placebo group. Encouraged by the results, the county has begun several more acupuncture detoxification projects.[2]

Al-Care, an outpatient substance abuse program in Albany, New York, treats a thousand clients a year with acupuncture. The clinic administration reports that their rate of inpatient referral for detoxification has dropped from 15 percent to 5 percent since acupuncture was added to the program. The rate of chronic relapse has dropped 40 percent in the same period.[3]

SLEEP TEA

The Lincoln Hospital Substance Abuse Program developed an herbal tea that helps addicts going through withdrawal. A form of this combination of herbs has been used in ancient cultures for thousands of years. Hebrew Watson says he continues to drink what he calls Sleep Tea, which helps him sleep and keep things in balance. The Lincoln mixture contains chamomile, peppermint, catnip, skullcap, hops, and yarrow, and it is sweetened using honey instead of sugar. The tea, according to Dr. Smith, is used to promote relaxation and treat insomnia. It is also effective in alcohol detoxification, if taken hourly. According to Dr. Smith, these herbs are not habit-forming and do not carry a risk of overdose or misuse.

Acupuncture and Jailed Addicts

Statistics are clear. Drug-related crimes are extremely high in this country, and the rate of repeat of illegal activities following release from corrections facilities is staggering. In 1988, Washington, D.C. Uniform Crime Statistics reported that 80 percent of the nation's capital's murders were drug-related. And in a survey of state and federal prisoners, more than 60 percent of those incarcerated used drugs on a regular basis before arrest. And although putting criminals in already overcrowded prisons keeps them clean and off the streets for a short period of time, without effective treatment, their drug problem will more than likely return. In an attempt to find solutions to this serious dilemma, city and state departments of corrections have been piloting acupuncture treatment programs.

According to a report from the Traditional Acupuncture Institute, which compiles statistics from acupuncture programs around the nation, the tab picked up by taxpayers for treating addicted criminals is dropping, while criminal activity and recidivism among ex-convicts is also decreasing, thanks in part to the adoption of acupuncture treatment by correctional institutions. Here are some of the findings of studies and information collected by the Traditional Acupuncture Institute:

- A 1994 California study reported that the cost of treating 150,000 drug abusers was $209 million. Benefits received in the first year after treatment added up to an estimated $1.5 billion in savings in terms of reduced crime.
- According to the California Drug and Alcohol Treatment Assessment Study compiled in 1994, criminal activity dropped by two-thirds following treatment.
- In the same 1994 California study, it was reported that for every dollar spent on alcohol and other drug treatment, taxpayers saved $7 in social costs.
- In 1993, a pilot program was established with the Baltimore Women's Detention Center in cooperation with the Traditional Acupuncture Institute and Johns Hopkins Hospital. Since the program's inception, more than 612 women have participated, with 95 percent completing the program. Corrections officials report that the inmates report feeling calmer and healthier, and that the inmates who have been treated are more cooperative with other inmates and guards.
- Drug Court, a Dade County, Florida, program, offers acupuncture treatment as an alternative to prison for felony drug offenders. Of fifty percent choosing to participate complete the year-long program.
- Oregon State law mandates that no one can enter a methadone treatment program without first attempting acupuncture treatment.

The Three-Tiered Protocol for Treating Addicted Convicts

The NADA and the National Association of Criminal Justice Planners released a recommended protocol for a three-tiered program for treating addicts. These suggestions have been widely accepted. The number of acupuncture treatments is tapered depending on the length of time that a person has remained sober. The first tier involves the most frequent acupuncture treatments. The three-tiered approach takes into account the understanding that the relapse is often part of recovery, so it is designed to help the patient progress at his or her own rate. If a patient relapses in the second stage, he or she is simply returned to the first stage, which offers more frequent acupuncture treatment. This approach, according to Hebrew Watson, is very helpful and it teaches the patients a sense of honesty, he says. "All they ask is that you tell the truth. If you use, you have to tell them so they can help you."

PORTLAND ADDICTIONS ACUPUNCTURE CENTER

Opening in 1991, the Portland center treats about 170 clients each week. According to information compiled by the Traditional Acupuncture Institute, Columbia, Maryland, the center reports that:

- Ninety percent of those who complete three months of addictions treatment at the center are drug-free three months later.
- The re-arrest rate for convicted felons who have completed the program is 3 percent, compared to 40–60 percent for felony drug abusers who do not have this type of treatment.
- Before acupuncture was added to Portland's treatment program, only 34 percent of the participants completed treatment. With the addition of acupuncture, 85 percent complete treatment.
- With the addition of acupuncture treatment, the recidivism rate after six months dropped by 20 percent.

Community Health Initiatives: The Penn North Neighborhood Center

In addition to acupuncture calming the mind so that the addict can better participate in his or her own recovery, the community networking component is a very important link in treatment programs that combine traditional and alternative approaches. And according to Raeford Ellison, the clinical director and program manager of the Penn North Neighborhood Center in Baltimore, creating possibilities for recovering addicts is a very important component of their treatment program. The community becomes part of the treatment process and, says Ellison, the neighborhood churches have been very helpful. Once the cravings are gone and the addict is clean, their life needs a great deal of repair. Some of the people have been homeless and haven't eaten for days. So getting a place to stay and something to eat may be the first step. Then other things follow during the five-phase components of the Penn North program. "Many of the people who come here, even if they are homeless, have a college education and we help them make new supportive connections. It makes a difference in their lives. It's about self esteem, learning who they are and supporting them in life." Sometimes it means helping them find clothes or shoes for a job interview or patching up things with their family or learning how to take care of their health. According to Ellison, the acupuncture treatment is a small part of the whole picture, it's not just an addictions problem. The addiction is just a symptom of a life problem, he says. "Sometimes we help bridge the gap to the community for the patient. With what we're doing at Penn North, everybody's life in this community will be touched in many ways."

But this time, he says that the people at the Penn North Neighborhood Center helped him learn about what was going on as he came down off heroin. He was also motivated to do some of his own research. "They are partners with you in your healing," says Hebrew about the Penn North approach to care. "They have taught me patience and to accept life on life's terms. Now when I go to NA [Narcotics Anonymous] meetings, I hear what people are saying. They also taught me about the different seasons the body goes through. That really helps me understand my own body."

Because Hebrew attributes some of his healing to the sense of community that is established at the clinic, he believes that it is now his duty to help others. And he does. Nearly every day he stops by the clinic to see if there are any newcomers. He'll sit down with them and share a piece of his own truth. Hebrew touches a spot in these troubled people that nonaddicts could never be able to reach.

Judging from his own recovery experience and those of the others he has helped, he believes that most of the time addicts want to stop but they aren't given the proper information and the right guidance in the process of recovery. He tells newcomers to the clinic that there's no miracle cure, that it's not a one-time thing. Quitting is an ongoing process that becomes a part of your life. "I tell them, the first few weeks just be quiet and listen." And then he softens, understanding some of their fears. "They can't take anything away from you. They can only add to what you have."

The Penn North Neighborhood Center, an outgrowth of the Traditional Acupuncture Institute's Community Health Initiative with the Baltimore Women's Detention Center, not only treats those seeking addictions treatment but others in the community with other health problems. It is this blending that Ellison says is important. A corporate grant from the ABLE Foundation of $150,000 got the neighborhood center operating and helps those unable to pay. Students and staff from the Traditional Acupuncture Institute volunteer their time to treat the patients at Penn North. According to the acupuncture institute's president, Robert Duggan, who volunteers with his wife, Susan, every Friday at the clinic, this is one of the most rewarding experiences. As he recounts the details of several success stories—the homeless crack-addicted mother, now clean and working, the alcoholic who needed shoes and learned how to care for his diabetes—his eyes sparkle, the love and concern evident.

TWELVE

Miracles: Prayer, Spirituality, Death, and Healing

"I think that during my first bout with cancer I found that in talking to traditional medicine doctors their attitudes were so bleak. They didn't allow much for miracles or the body's ability to heal itself."

—Elizabeth Zintle, lung cancer patient, who died in February 1997

PRAYER

Studies show that a great number of Americans turn to prayer in times of crisis. Each year more than 4 million people travel to the healing waters of Lourdes in France, and a million or so more to Medjugorje in Bosnia-Herzegovina. Organized religions collect the tales of the unexplained: the lame child who walked, the blind man who saw, and the dead Lazarus who came to life. So why do we have such difficulty acknowledging miracles as an important part of healing? For the skeptics, it's the whole idea that something cannot be explained that gets them going. (Studies are starting to dispute the idea that miracles can't be explained.) And for doctors and scientists who want to believe, recognizing that such phenomena occur puts their professional standing in jeopardy. Believing in miracles is a stigma for doctors. When Bernie Siegel, M.D., the surgeon, was transformed into Bernie Siegel, M.D., the patient guide, he faced incredible scrutiny from his peers. Yet he says that he saw too many miracles not to believe. His colleagues shunned him. Another surgeon shared a similar experience. He was well respected and had a lucrative practice, but once he began talking about miracles, prayer, and connecting with the patient, colleagues he had known for years avoided him at all costs. They'd walk on the other side of the hall or turn down another corridor to make certain he got the message that what he was doing wasn't acceptable.

Siegel and other visionaries are just a beat ahead of their time. They've always been viewed by the mainstream as crazy, delusional, but their ideas, originally scoffed at, rise to prominence in time. Take radio's inventor, Guglielmo Marconi, who was hospitalized as insane when he shared his ideas about transmitting information across invisible waves through space. Or Johannes Kepler, who talked about the pull of lunar gravity. He was considered mad. Yet we eventually had to see that these madmen had uncovered truth. We turn on the radio without question. We teach Kepler's theories in the classroom. Perhaps in another ten years the prayerful aspect of healing will be just as commonplace. We're in an age of transition, and the believers, like Bernie Siegel, Larry Dossey, Pali DeLevitt, Sandra McLanahan, Peter Bower, Jody Forman, Caroline Jaffe, Bob Duggan, and Larry LeShan, among others, continue to make their ideas known, even in the face of scrutiny.

> *"As Christians in a healing ministry for more than sixteen years, we know that it is the power of Jesus Christ working through us that heals. We do not claim that any power of our own heals, but we have seen and experienced too many healings in our ministry to doubt that the power is there."*
>
> —Father Peter McCall and Maryanne Lacy,
> cofounders of the House of Peace, the Bronx,
> and the authors of *Rise and Be Healed.*

For some people, the idea of prayer and healing are an important aspect of their religious practices. Healing comes from a saint, from Mary, or from God. But as studies have shown, spiritual, prayer-based healing is universal, and no one religion has a monopoly on healing. It occurs with regularity in Eastern and Western belief systems as well as in more nature or spirit-based practices. It appears that the unifying principles—love, compassion, a sense of oneness and empathy—transcend dogma or religious boundaries.

"The miracle comes quietly into the mind that stops an instant and is still. It reaches gently from that quiet time, and from the mind it healed in quiet then, to other minds to share its quietness."

Choose Once Again, Selections from
A Course in Miracles

STUDIES ON PRAYER AND DISTANT HEALING

In the past few years, hundreds of clinical studies point to the positive effects of distance healing. But the first studies on the effects of prayer on health date back to the nineteenth century. Sir Francis Galton attempted to assess the longevity of individuals who were frequently prayed for, such as priests, heads of state, and monarchs. Although his research concluded that there was no appreciable effect, and his studies were flawed, he created an environment in which it made sense to begin to consider the correlation between the two. And since Galton's early attempts, many published reports indicate that people were able to influence cellular and biological systems through prayer or through nonlocal mental means. Psychologist William G. Braud summarizes this research:

"There exist many published reports of experiments in which persons were able to influence a variety of cellular and other biological systems through mental means. The target systems for these investigations have included bacteria, yeast, fungi, mobile algae, plants, protozoa, larvae, insects, chicks, mice, rats, gerbils, cats, and dogs, as well as cellular preparations and enzyme activities. In human target persons, eye movements, muscular movements, electrodermal activity, plethysmographis activity, respiration, and brain rhythms have been affected through direct mental influence."[1]

As Braud observes, these studies have shown that individuals from a distance could actually influence the physiological functions of living organisms, even when the receiver of the prayerfulness was not aware of the activity. And although some of the studies did not name a particular religion or prayer that healers used, all of the healing situations involved prayerfulness, or feelings of compassion, genuine caring, love, or empathy with the receiver.

In the mid-1980s a California cardiologist, Dr. Randolph Byrd, gathered a group of born-again Christians to pray as part of a study of 393 heart patients. According to the *Southern Medical Journal,* the group of patients who were prayed for developed less cases of accumulated fluid in the lungs, a result of coronary problems, and required fewer antibiotics. None of the group who were prayed for required breathing assistance, whereas 12 in the group who were not prayed for did.

Two researchers, David B. Larson and Susan S. Larson, surveyed all the issues of the *American Journal of Psychiatry* and the *Archives of General Psychiatry* for a twelve-year period. They discovered that 92 percent of the studies measuring participation in religious ceremony, social support, prayer, and relationship with God showed a mental health benefit.[2]

More Studies on the Effect of Prayer on Healing

- Psychiatry researchers at the University of California at San Francisco are studying the effects of distant prayer on AIDS patients in a controlled study, . Twenty praying healers from New York and Washington, D.C., are part of the study, sending healing messages or intentions to individuals with advanced AIDS in California. The researchers are looking for changes in T-cell counts to determine whether prayer affects immunity.
- A National Institutes of Health study is examining the efficacy of prayer on substance abuse patients. The NIH study has come under scrutiny by the Freedom from Religion Foundation, an atheist group, saying that taxpayer dollars should not be used for this type of study.
- Physicians at Temple University are studying the effects of prayer on 150 infants at risk of dying from neonatal conditions.
- University of Arkansas researchers are looking at the response of muscle cells to distant prayer.

As more and more cases of distant healing are recorded, there are many implications for how we will look at medicine and health care in the future. The distant prayer model of healing might serve to create new foundations. According to Larry Dossey, there have been three eras of health care in this country: the first being in the mid-1800s when medicine became mechanistic; the second in the 1950s, when the concept of mind/body medicine came into play; and now we are at the beginning of the third era of nonlocal medicine. But, as

Dossey points out, all three eras are important and overlap. The way he views medicine's future, the three eras will be interwoven into one seamless therapeutic fabric.

> *"Of course it was not I who cured. It was power from the outer world, and the visions and ceremonies had only made me like a hole through which the power would come to the two-leggeds. If I thought I was doing it myself, the hole would close up and no power would come through it."*
>
> —Black Elk, Oglala Sioux

SPIRITUAL HEALERS AND THE SACRED CONTRACT

Back in 1966, psychologist Larry LeShan investigated the correlation between psychological states and cancer. And in his efforts, this pioneering thinker discovered that there were two types of spiritual healing: Type I and Type II. In the first type of healing, the healer seeks to become one with the patient, so that when the healer enters a prayerful state, the two become as one with God or the universe. Such healers do not try to do anything to the patient and do not require physical contact. Conversely, Type II healers must be present with the patient, and touch is part of the healing interaction. These healers talk about the flow of energy through the healer's hands. Both patients and healers describe feelings of heat emanating from the hands to the patient's body. Among Type II healers, some see themselves as causing the healing power, while others see themselves as the vehicle for transmitting the healing energy. Following his early studies, LeShan considered Type I healing the more prevalent and important.

Finding Oneness: The Sacred Contract

Perhaps the loving journey between two is the journey to healing. Does the journey of the two become the journey of one? In ancient times, the great healers, the shamans, were only able to heal after spiritual quests of oneness. "Healers have to be impeccable on every level," says Pali DeLevitt, Ph.D, of the University of Virginia Medical School faculty." A shaman didn't declare that he was a healer. The community acknowledges the spiritual and healership of that person. They have a sense of joy. A quality of love and compassion and an ability to facilitate healing. But everybody heals the self." Pali calls this relationship the sacred contract between the healer and the patient; between the patient and the self; and between the healer and the healee and the universe.

> *"For where two or three are gathered together in My name,*
> *I am there in the midst of them."*
>
> —Matthew 18: 20

QUANTUM PHYSICS

As scientists try to find a reason behind spiritual healing, theories continue to surface. The quantum physics theory seems to be getting more attention from scientists. Several scientific experiments have shown that once two electrons have had contact, when one changes the other changes immediately, even when the two are separated by great distance. These changes do not require the transmission of energy, and their connection does not lessen with distance—a concept very similar to prayerful distance healing relationships.

STUDIES ON HEALING IN COMMUNITY

An acupuncturist shared with me that he believes this country's violence and crime is directly related to our lack of community with others. And studies indicate that people living in isolation die sooner, get sicker, and often suffer more from chronic conditions.

In the early 1960s researchers found a little Italian community in Roseto, Pennsylvania where the rates of death from heart disease and other conditions were significantly lower than the national averages. Researchers wanted to find out their secret. The people of Roseto smoked, they ate many of the wrong foods, and didn't get enough exercise. So what was it that made the difference? It was a strong sense of community and family ties. Interestingly, when the younger children set sail for new frontiers and severed community connections, mortality rates in Roseto soon paralleled national statistics.

Researchers at the University of Michigan found a definitive link between isolation and a lack of social relationships and poor health. According to researchers, the 10–20 percent of people who claim they have no one to share their inner feelings with, or who come into contact with others less than once a week, are at the greatest risk of disease. And compared to their more social counterparts, their risk of dying increases in some cases by 300 percent.

Stanford Medical School psychiatrists, led by Dr. David Speigel, discovered that breast cancer patients who joined support groups lived nearly twice as long as those who received only medical care.

> *"Healing is the filling-in of the hidden areas of a person's life that are leading that person away from their full experience of health. So healing involves bringing these areas into consciousness and transforming them. Often in the process a physical cure takes place, but not always, and therefore there needs to be a distinction between curing and healing. We can often cure through surgery and drugs, which simply means cutting out the affected part, or removing the symptoms through pharmaceutical or even nutritional means. Ultimately, however, this will not effect a complete cure until the emotional, psychological, and spiritual aspects of the condition are also addressed."*
>
> —Christiane Northrup, M.D.

HEALING IN DEATH

In our country we shun our old and our terminally ill. We warehouse them into nursing homes, leaving them to die alone. According to the *New England Journal of Medicine*, out of 400 patients, 350 die alone. And we often forget that there is a person underneath that crumpled body. It is a person that can love and be loved just for who he or she is. I remember Naomi. She was a beautiful woman in her seventies. And she had cancer. But that didn't change the fact that she loved the theater and loved the life she knew would soon be over. She had been put in a nursing home by her family to die. No one visited her. I would stop by and spend some time with her. It all started when she said she wanted to analyze my handwriting, and, of course, that piqued my interest. We laughed and talked, and one Sunday we took a trip to the theater in Philadelphia. The trip was hard on her, but at the same time it was wonderful for both of us. I watched her great spirit. Her sense of knowing it was her time to travel from her physical body to the light of lights. In our brief encounter, Naomi taught me many things.

"It is in this arena that you will see the spiritual truth. I talk to people at the point of dying, and they hear music, they see angels, they see figures in the room. It happens all the time. A lot of what we do in alternative medicine is to help us live and die gracefully."

—Sandra McLanahan, M.D.

AFTERWORD

Where Do We Go from Here?

"It is clear that we are moving from a world in which we look to experts in healthcare to make decisions for us to a world in which we have recovered our ability, as individuals, families, and communities, to heal ourselves and to make the advice and skills of the 'experts' supplemental to our reliance on the innate human ability to heal."

—Robert Duggan, MAc, MA, DiplAc
president and cofounder, Traditional Acupuncture
Institute, Columbia, MD.

There's no doubt about it, the way we view health care in this country is changing. The sheer momentum of the general consumer's search for something different is forcing the conventional Western medical community to stand up and listen. And it's not that anyone is proposing throwing all our country's medical advances out the window in favor of alternatives, but what we're looking for is more, and in a sense, less: less drugs, less surgery, less invasive procedures, less expense, less testing; more listening, more personal attention, more natural options, more education, and more love. So we're asking, How can the best of a technologically advanced medical culture and the best of ancient traditional medicine work in tandem? On the surface, it seems fairly simple. Take what we do best and what alternative medicine and traditional Eastern medicine do best, and integrate the two. But in the current climate, the transition will not be that easy. There are laws and regulations that keep it from happening. There are researchers and doctors who keep it from happening, and there are alternative practitioners who keep it from happening. And we keep it from happening. Everyone has a part to play in the building up and the tearing down of the barriers to an integrated system of care in this country.

THE PERILS OF MAINSTREAMING ALTERNATIVE MEDICINE

At the present time, alternatives, which are actually traditional methods of care, remain on the periphery of society, and practitioners from the East and West struggle with the next steps. And the very values and principles that make alternatives appealing to us—the extra time and attention paid to us by practitioners, the person-to-person contact and understanding, the heart of healing—could be lost if we mainstream these therapies into an existing system that is dictated by the dollar. Insurers and managed care companies could mandate the amount of time allotted to each patient, just as they have with conventional doctors. Instead of two hours, we might get five minutes. This would only serve to add one more less expensive therapy into the Western arsenal of cures. And we as patients would remain unsatisfied. Alternative practitioners, if mainstreamed into the current hierarchy of the medical model, would be relegated to a subservient position under Western medical doctors. Rather than working side-by-side in their respective philosophies, they would be forced into a paraprofessional role, leaving Western doctors with the final approval in a power-based model. We'd rather avoid such a scenario. Perhaps the greatest peril of all would be that alternative practitioners would join the Western medical model paradigm that views natural life processes as failures and problems. Currently, pain and death are failures, as far as Western physicians are concerned. How can this be? Since the beginning of time, in the natural course of things, we all feel pain and we will all die.

BEING REALISTIC ABOUT RESEARCH

Many researchers have offered alternatives to the rigid double-blind, placebo-controlled studies that our country is demanding occur for alternative treatments and herbal remedies. But no one is budging. Not all the Western therapies that are commonly prescribed have gone through this type of testing. And a great majority of Eastern remedies have no known harmful side effects. So why are we creating such an impossible standard? A standard of testing that does not even apply in many cases to the philosophies of Eastern prescription. We are attempting to study the efficacy of one herb for a particular disease, yet Eastern practitioners generally never prescribe one herb; a combination is prepared. According to Eastern medical theory, every person's diagnosis is individual, and there are many variables that are weighed in prescribing treatment. In double-blind, placebo-controlled trials, this mode of treatment cannot be accommodated, and therefore the information obtained from a multimillion dollar study will not tell us anything about the Eastern mode of treatment. As consumers, we need to ask why these extensive studies, many of which have already been conducted in other countries, must occur again. And why can't the findings from foreign researchers serve as proof of the efficacy of a particular herbal medication or therapy? Why must we allocate billions of dollars to do what has already been done? Interestingly, when I started researching current studies for this book, I contacted several of the NIH-appointed research centers for alternative medicine. And because of the administrative controls that have been established for studies, the first year of funding was just to get the study protocol in place. In the second and third years, ten or twenty people would be studied. So several million dollars later we'll know how a certain therapy or herbal preparation affected ten or twenty people? What got us in this situation? How can we make studies more realistic and down to earth? We need to ask those in power these questions and demand that our dollars be spent more effectively.

STATE-SPONSORED CHANGES

We have a long way to go in making alternative treatments more accessible to more people, although some states such as California, New Mexico, and Washington are mandating insurance coverage of alternative therapies, and licensing is bringing alternative practitioners into a more equal status with their Western counterparts. Yet there are many states that are keeping Eastern practitioners under the thumb of Western medical bureaucracy. Take Virginia, for example. I would like to go to an acupuncturist for diagnosis and treatment. To do this, I must first go to a Western medical doctor for a referral to a service that I must pay for out of my pocket. The visit to the conventional Western doctor will be paid for by my insurance. Currently, thirty-three states and the District of Columbia license and recognize acupuncturists. Three states mandate insurance coverage for acupuncture and four states require that plans pay for Western doctors trained as acupuncturists. According to available statistics, acupuncturists have about

$500 million in business with an average of nine to twelve patient visits per year.

FINDING THE PATH TO THE FUTURE

For any dramatic recovery, a change in thinking must occur. This paradigm shift is currently leading us in new directions. We as health care consumers must stop thinking that we are sick and learn how to be well. A health care practitioner's success should be measured by how many patients stay well, not by how many come in sick. We need to learn how to care for our bodies—how to limit stress, do more of what we love, find our spiritual center, stop isolating ourselves, and begin loving, eating better, and getting rid of risky behaviors that will eventually make us sick. In many ways it is up to us to set the path for the future. And it is in setting this path that the regulations and laws will follow. More important, in these changes perhaps we will discover that the secret of healing lies within each of us. And when we discover this secret, we will begin to listen to the natural cycles of living. We will honor our life for what we believe is important. We will journey on the same path as ancient cultures, and on this pilgrimage we will find the truth, the love, and the light of the universe. It is on this path that we set for ourselves and our children and grandchildren that we will find healing. In life and in death, we will be healed.

NOTES

CHAPTER I

1. This parasitic disease occurs most frequently in tropical countries and is often acquired from bathing in infested lakes and rivers. The eggs from three species of flukes provoke inflammatory reactions in the bladder, intestinal walls, or liver. Today this disease still afflicts more than 200 million people worldwide.
2. Charles B. Clayman, ed., *The American Medical Association Encyclopedia of Medicine* (New York: Random House, 1989).
3. *Chinese Civilization: A Sourcebook*, 2d ed. (New York: Free Press, 1993), 77–79.
4. Jeanne Rose, "A History of Herbs and Herbalism," in *American Herbalism*, ed. Michael Tierra, (Freedom, Calif.: The Crossing Press , 1992).
5. *Chinese Civilization: A Sourcebook*, 2d ed.
6. Ibid.
7. Kathryn S. Brown, "Looking Back at Jenner, Vaccine Developers Prepare for Twenty-First Century," *The Scientist 10*, no. 7, (April 1996): 14–17.
8. Ibid.
9. Ibid.
10. *Alternative Medicine: Expanding Medical Horizons* A Report to the National Institutes of Health on Alternative Medical Systems and Practices in the United States. (Washington, D.C.: U.S. Government Printing Office, 1994), NIH Publication No. 94-066.
11. Ibid.
12. Ibid.

13. Taken from the *Archives of Internal Medicine* 155 (CITY: University of Arizona, 1995).
14. Ibid.
15. National Institutes of Health Office of Alternative Medicine "Complementary and Alternative Medicine at the NIH," , 3, no. 5 (October 1996).

CHAPTER 2

1. Daniel Reid, *The Complete Book of Chinese Health and Healing* (Boston: Shambhala, 1995).
2. Michael O. Smith, *Acupuncture Treatment for Alcoholism* (National Acupuncture Detoxification Association Inc., 1986).

CHAPTER 3

1. Michael O. Smith, *Acupuncture Treatment for Alcoholism* (National Acupuncture Detoxification Association Inc., 1986).

CHAPTER 4

1. Howard Moffet, "Using Acupuncture and Herbs for the Treatment of HIV Infection," American College of Traditional Chinese Medicine Experience, AIDS Patient Care, *A Journal for Health Care Professionals*, August 1994, 194-198.
2. Ibid.
3. Howard Moffet, "Using Acupuncture and Herbs for the Treatment of HIV Infection," American College of Traditional Chinese Medicine Experience, AIDS Patient Care, August 1994, 194-98.
4. M. Goh, "Acupuncture Treatment for Neuropathy—Patients with HIV Infection," International Symposium on Viral Hepatitis and AIDS, Beijing, April 1991.
5. Lu Weibo et al., "Clinical Observation on Treating 112 HIV/AIDS Patients with Glyke," International Conference on STD, Yokohama, August 1994.
6. Leanna J. Standish, Principal Investigator, "Alternative Medicine in HIV/AIDS: Current State of the Science and Justification for Research," Bastyr University AIDS Research Center, Seattle, Washington, June 1996.
7. Ibid.
8. Ibid.
9. Beth Reinhard, "Patients Find New Hope in Unconventional Study,"

West Palm Beach Post, February 18, 1996, 17A.

10. Jin Lin Wang, "Chinese Herbs and Acupuncture to Treat ARC and AIDS," Oriental Medical Center, Los Angeles, 1988.

11. Ibid.

12. Sheila McNamara, *Traditional Chinese Medicine*, (New York: Basic Books, a Division of Harper Collins, 1996).

13. U.S. Congress Office of Technological Assessment. *Unconventional Cancer Treatments, Behavioral and Psychological Approaches*, OTA H-405, (Washington, D.C.: U.S. Government Printing Office, September 1990).

14. Ibid.

CHAPTER 5

1. "Mind-Body Interventions", *Alternative Medicine: Expanding Medical Horizons,* A Report to the National Institutes of Health on Alternative Medical Systems and Practices in the United States. (Washington, D.C.: U.S. Government Printing Office, 1994), NIH Publication No. 94-066.

2. E. L. Idler and S. Kasl, "Health Perceptions and Survival: Do Global Evaluations of Health Status Really Predict Mortality?" *Journal of Gerontology* 46 (1991): S55–S65.

3. Claire Cassidy, *Social Science Theory and Methods*, Traditional Acupuncture Institute, (Columbia, MD: 1996).

CHAPTER 6

1. *Alternative Medicine: Expanding Medical Horizons*, A Report to the National Institutes of Health on Alternative Medical Systems and Practices in the United States. (Washington, D.C.: U.S. Government Printing Office, 1994), NIH Publication No. 94–066, p. 4.

2. Judith Mandelbaum-Schmid, "Prophets and Pioneers," *Self*, (November 1996): 167.

3. *Alternative Medicine: Expanding Medical Horizons*, A Report to the National Institutes of Health on Alternative Medical Systems and Practices in the United States. (Washington, D.C.: Government Printing Office, 1994), NIH Publication No. 94–066, p. 17.

4. Ibid., 17.

5. Ibid., 321–322.

6. Ibid., 14.

7. Ibid., 15.

CHAPTER 7

1. T. Colin Campbell and Christine Cox, *The China Project: Keys to Better Health, Discovered In Our Living Laboratory,* (Ithaca, N.Y.: New Century Nutrition, 1996).

2. Ibid
3. Ibid.
4. Ibid.
5. Ibid.
6. Ibid.
7. Ibid.
8. Ibid.
9. Ibid.
10. Ibid.
11. Ibid.
12. Ibid.

CHAPTER 8

1. David G. Spoerke, Jr. *Herbal Medications* (Santa Barbara, Calif.: Woodbridge Press, 1980).
2. Ibid.
3. *Alternative Medicine: Expanding Medical Horizons,* A Report to the National Institutes of Health on Alternative Medical Systems and Practices in the United States. (Washington D.C.: U.S. Government Printing Office, 1994), NIH Publication N0. 94-006.
4. U.S. Congress, Office of Technological Assessment. *Unconventional Cancer Treatments, Herbal Treatments,* OTA H-405, Washington, D.C. U.S. Government Printing Office, September 1990.

General information on herbs in this chapter comes from the following publications, which are listed in the references section: Michael Tierra, *American Herbalism*; Jean Carper, Food: *Your Miracle Medicine*; Earl Mindell, *Earl Mindell's Herb Bible*; Robert Sachs, *Health for Life, Secrets of Tibetan Ayurveda*; and David G. Spoerke, *Herbal Medications*.

CHAPTER 10

1. The Effects of Tai Chi on Balance-Impaired Subjects, Rebecca Phalen MPT, Deborah Hartford, MPT, Diane Wrisley PT, NCS, Lawrence Mann, 1997.
2. This summary of preliminary study information on qigong was taken from "A Medical Assessment of Qigong," by Lao Cen, Beijing.

CHAPTER 11

1. Testimony from Michael O. Smith, M.D., Director, Substance Abuse Division, Department of Psychiatry of Lincoln Hospital, New York City, to the National Institutes of Health, Office of Alternative Medicine, and the National Wellness Coalition.
2. Michael O. Smith, *Acupuncture Treatment for Alcoholism*, (National Acupuncture Detoxification Association Inc., 1986).
3. Taken from an interview with Michael Smith and from Traditional Acupuncture Institute information.
4. Testimony from Michael O. Smith, M.D., Director, Substance Abuse Division, Department of Psychiatry of Lincoln Hospital, New York City, to the National Institutes of Health, Office of Alternative Medicine, and the National Wellness Coalition.

CHAPTER 12

1. W.G. Braud, "Human Interconnectedness; Research Indications," *ReVision* 14: 140–48.
2. *Alternative Medicine: Expanding Medical Horizons,* A Report to the National Institutes of Health on Alternative Medical Systems and Practices in the United States (Washington, D.C.: U.S. Government Printing Office, 1994), NIH Publication No. 94-066.

REFERENCES

In addition to the hundreds of interviews with alternative practitioners, Western medical doctors, patients, families of patients, insurers, government officials, scientists, researchers, anthropologists, believers, and nonbelievers, the following sources were used. Specific studies are referenced in each chapter.

ARTICLES AND MEETINGS

Baker, Lucille M. "Still Catching Sunbeams." *OT Week,* August 29, 1991.

Beinfield, Harriet, and Efrem Korngold. "Chinese Traditional Medicine: An Introductory Overview." *Alternative Therapies* 1, no. 1 (March 1995).

Brown, Ellen. "Alternative Medicine Converts its Skeptics." *Managed Healthcare* (June 1996).

Duggan, Bob. "Complementary Medicine: Transforming Influence or Footnote to History?" *Alternative Therapies,* no. 2 (May 1995).

———. "Complementary Medicine: Transforming Influence or Footnote to History?" *Alternative Therapies* 1, no. 2 (May 1995).

———. "Alternative Medicine Offers Sensible Options in Health Care." *Seattle Post-Intelligencer,* May 9, 1996.

Goss, Kathy. "Qigong for Health: New Instructional Video in Ancient Chinese Healing Exercises." Horizontes No. 12, March 22, 1996.

Langone, John. "Challenging the Mainstream." *Time,* Fall 1996.

Lovette, Martha. "Qigong for Health: It's Good for Everybody." *The Noe Review,* Summer 1996.

Mandelbaum-Schmid, Judith. "Prophets and Pioneers." *SELF,* November 1996, p. 167.

Moffet, Howard. "Using Acupuncture and Herbs for the Treatment of HIV Infection." *AIDS Patient Care* (August 1994).

Pereira, Joseph. "The Healing Power of Prayer Is Tested by Science." *Wall Street Journal,* December 20, 1995.

Phalen, Kathleen. "Second Chance at Life." *Reading Eagle/Reading Times,* February 25, 1995.

Phalen, Kathleen. "Fat Nearly Killed Him." *Reading Eagle/Reading Times,*

Phalen, Kathleen. "Pinpointing a Treatment." *Reading Eagle/Reading Times,* 1995.

Phalen, Kathleen. "Plaintalk: How to Get the Most from Your Trip to the Doctor." *Reading Eagle/Reading Times,* February 7, 1995.

Phalen, Kathleen. "Partners in the Exam Room." *Reading Eagle/ Reading Times,* February 7, 1995.

Philip, Tom. "The Modern Fight Against AIDS Turns to Ancient Weapons." *Sacramento Bee,* October 6, 1996.

Reinhard, Beth. "Patients Find New Hope in Unconventional Study." *West Palm Beach Post,* February 18, 1996.

Weber, David O. "The Mainstreaming of Alternative Medicine." *Healthcare Forum Journal,* (November/December 1996).

Weibo, Lu. "Treatment of AIDS by Traditional Chinese Medicine and Materia Medica." *Journal of Traditional Chinese Medicine* 11, no. 4 (1991).

Whitaker, Barbara. "Now in the HMO: Yoga Teachers and Naturopaths." *New York Times,* November 24, 1996.

The New American Medicine Series of Articles: "The Promise of Energy Healing," Helen Caldicott. "Prophets and Pioneers," Judith Mandelbaum-Schmid. "It's Superplant!," Jillian Mackenzie. "5 Perfect Moves," Terry Doyle. "Best of Both Worlds," Mary Alice Kellog. "Is the New Medicine Right for You?," Mary Alice Kellogg. "East Meets Beast," Katharine Greider. SELF, November 1996.

"T'ai-Chi Ch'uan Research Abstracts," compiled by Tricia Yu, 1996.

"Alternative Health Care Providers: Gaining Ground in State Legislatures." *State Health Notes,* November 25, 1996.

The Effects of Tai Chi on Balance-Impaired Subjects, Rebecca Phalen, MPT, Deborah Hartford, MPT, Diane Wrisley PT, NCS, Lawrence Mann, 1997.

BOOKS/PUBLICATIONS

U.S. Congress Office of Technological Assessment. *Unconventional Cancer Treatments.* OTA H-405. Washington, D.C.: U.S. Government Printing Office, September 1990.

The Chinese Way to a Long and Healthy Life. Beijing: The People's Medical Publishing House of Beijing; New York: Hippocrene Books, 1984.

Carper, Jean. *Food: Your Miracle Medicine.* New York: Harper Perennial, 1994.

Clayman, Charles B. *The American Medical Association Encyclopedia of Medicine.* New York: Random House, 1989.

Connelly, Diane M. *Traditional Acupuncture: The Law of the Five Elements.* 1994.

Levine, Stephen. *A Gradual Awakening.* New York: Anchor Books/ Doubleday, 1989.

Liu, Yanchi. *The Essential Book of Traditional Chinese Medicine.* New York: Columbia University Press, 1988.

McNamara, Sheila. *Traditional Chinese Medicine.* New York: Basic Books, 1996.

Mindell, Earl. *Earl Mindell's Herb Bible.* New York: Simon and Schuster, 1992.

Porkert, Manfred, and Christian Ullman. *Chinese Medicine.* New York: William Morrow and Company, 1982.

Sachs, Robert. *Health for Life, Secrets of Tibetan Ayurveda.* Santa Fe: Clear Light Publishers, 1995.

Skocpol, Theda. *Boomerang.* New York: W. W. Norton, 1996.

Spoerke, David G. *Herbal Medications.* Santa Barbara, Calif.: Woodbridge Press Publishing Company, 1980.

Tierra, Michael. *American Herbalism.* Freedom, Calif: The Crossing Press, 1992.

Wolfe, Sidney M., M.D. *Women's Health Alert.* Reading, Mass.: Addison-Wesley, 1991.

Alternative Medicine: Expanding Medical Horizons. Washington, D.C.: U.S. Government Printing Office, 1994.

Weibo Lu, et al. "Clinical Observation on Treating 112 HIV/AIDS Patients with Glyke." International Conference on STD, Yokohama, August 1994.

Goh, M. "Acupuncture Treatment for Neuropathy—Patients with HIV International Symposium on Viral Hepatitis and AIDS, Beijing, April 1991.

Eisenberg, D. M. R. C. Kessler, C. Foster, F. E. Norlock, D.R. Calkins, and T. L. Delbanco. "Unconventional Medicine in the United States." *New England Journal of Medicine,* 328: (1993) 246-252.

"Acupuncture Treatment for Alcoholism," Michael O. Smith, National Acupuncture Detoxification Association Inc., 1986.

Idler, E. L. and S. Kasl. "Health Perceptions and Survival: Do Global Evaluations of Health Status Really Predict Mortality?" *Journal of Gerontology.* 46(1991): S55–S65.

INDEX